Faith Community Nursing

3rd Edition

Scope and Standards of Practice

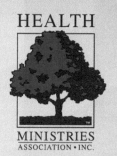

HEALTH
MINISTRIES
ASSOCIATION • INC.

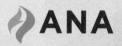

American Nurses Association
Silver Spring, Maryland 2017

Published by
American Nurses Association
8515 Georgia Avenue, Suite 400
Silver Spring, MD 20910-3492
1-800-274-4ANA
http://www.Nursingworld.org

The American Nurses Association (ANA) is the premier organization representing the interests of the nation's 3.6 million registered nurses. ANA advances the nursing profession by fostering high standards of nursing practice, promoting a safe and ethical work environment, bolstering the health and wellness of nurses, and advocating on health care issues that affect nurses and the public. ANA is at the forefront of improving the quality of health care for all.

The American Nurses Association (ANA) and the Health Ministries Association (HMA) are national professional associations. This ANA–HMA publication, *Faith Community Nursing: Scope and Standards of Practice, 3rd Edition*, reflects the thinking of the nursing profession on various issues and should be reviewed in conjunction with state board of nursing policies and practices. State law, rules, and regulations govern the practice of nursing, while *Faith Community Nursing: Scope and Standards of Practice, 3rd Edition* guides nurses in the application of their professional knowledge, skills, and responsibilities. For more about HMA, see pg. xii.

Notice

No responsibility is assumed by the publishers for any injury and/or damage to persons or property as a matter of products liability, negligence, or otherwise, or from any use or operation of any methods, products, instructions, or ideas contained in the material herein. Because of rapid advances in the medical sciences, in particular, independent verification of diagnoses and drug dosages should be made.

Library of Congress Cataloging-in-Publication Data

Names: American Nurses Association, issuing body. | Health Ministries Association.
Title: Faith community nursing : scope and standards of practice.
Description: Third edition. | Silver Spring, MD : American Nurses Association, 2017. |
Includes bibliographical references and index.
Identifiers: LCCN 2017032786 (print) | LCCN 2017032988 (ebook) |
ISBN 9780972608848 (ePDF) | ISBN 9780972608855 (ePub) |
ISBN 9780976821311 (Prc) | ISBN 9780972608831 (pbk. : alk. paper)
Subjects: | MESH: Parish Nursing--standards | Holistic Nursing--standards |
Nursing Process--standards | Practice Guideline
Classification: LCC RT120.P37 (ebook) | LCC RT120.P37 (print) | NLM WY 86.5 |
DDC 610.73/43--dc23
LC record available at https://lccn.loc.gov/2017032786

ISBN-13: 978-0-9726088-3-1   SAN: 851-3481   08/2017
First printing: August 2017

Contents

Contributors

For continuity and consistency, *Nursing: Scope and Standards of Practice, Third Edition*, was used as the template for developing this third edition of *Faith Community Nursing: Scope and Standards of Practice*. The volunteer workgroup used monthly conference calls and electronic communications to review, revise, and refine the scope and standards of faith community nursing. Fourteen practicing faith community nurses representing different areas of the country and various roles in this specialty practice contributed to this work. These contributors have active memberships in Health Ministries Association, American Nurses Association (ANA), Sigma Theta Tau, ANA-affiliated state nursing associations and faith community nursing councils or special interest groups, and Faith Community Nursing International. They hold leadership positions in multiple faith denominations' national health ministry organizations and networks. They actively partner with community organizations like the American Heart Association, the American Red Cross, and governmental health organizations such as the Health and Human Services Center for Faith-Based and Neighborhood Partnerships and the Centers for Medicare and Medicaid Services.

Faith Community Nursing Scope and Standards of Practice, Third Edition, is the product of a three-step review process. The first review process was a 30-day public comment period. The workgroup carefully considered all comments received for refinement of the document. The next step in the development process was evaluation by the ANA Committee on Nursing Practice Standards and final review and approval by the ANA Board of Directors. As a result, this document provides a national perspective on the current practice of this specialty of faith community nursing.

Faith Community Nursing Scope and Standards Workgroup, 2015–2017

Alyson J. Breisch, MSN, RN-BC
Faith Community Nurse and Commissioned Minister for
Congregational Health, United Church, Chapel Hill, North Carolina;
Proprietor, Breisch Health Education, PLLC; Chair, Faith Community
Nursing Scope and Standards of Practice Work Group, 2015–2017

Ms. Breisch has over 40 years' experience in nursing, 15 years in advanced practice nursing and 17 years' experience in faith community nursing. She directed a graduate nursing degree program in Health and Nursing Ministries and developed a continuing education curriculum for faith community nursing. She served as Director of Practice and Education on the Health Ministries Association Board of Directors from 2006 to 2014. She is a national consultant to healthcare systems and denominations on faith community nursing practice. She achieved American Nurses Credentialing Center certification by portfolio in Faith Community Nursing in 2015.

Nancy L. Rago-Durbin, MS, BSN, RN-BC
Director, Faith Community Nurse Ministry & Faith Community Nurse
Support Network Advocate Health Care, Downers Grove, Illinois

With more than 25 years of experience in health ministry, Nancy Durbin has been a leader in developing resources for faith community nursing that include policies, procedures, competencies, program evaluation, data measurement, and faith community nursing curriculum review. She currently serves as Director, Faith Community Nurse Constituents, chair of HMA Faith Community Nurse Mentor Program and HMA Faith Community Nursing Society for the Health Ministries Association, Inc. She has presented locally, nationally and internationally on the specialty practice of faith community nursing. She achieved American Nurses Credentialing Center certification by portfolio in Faith Community Nursing in 2014.

Marlene Feagan, MA, BSN, RN-BC
Health Ministries Coordinator, St. Elizabeth Healthcare,
Northern, Kentucky

Ms. Feagan has more than 30 years of nursing experience in critical care, behavioral health, chemical dependency, and faith community nursing. In 1997, Marlene developed and implemented a health ministries program as part of the continuum of care and community outreach serving faith communities and the community-at-large. She serves as president of the Health Ministries Association. She has been a national leader in advancing the professional role of faith community nursing. She provided leadership in the American Nurses Credentialing Center (ANCC) and Health Ministries Association partnership to develop the certification process for the specialty. She achieved ANCC certification by portfolio in Faith Community Nursing in 2014.

Karen Lynne Golie, BSN, RN
Supervisor, Faith Community Health Ministry, Carolinas HealthCare System, Charlotte, NC

Ms. Golie served as a faith community nurse. She has worked with the Carolinas HealthCare System's Faith Community Health Ministry program for 10 years as program education coordinator and currently as supervisor. Her work includes educational programming for community and staff and development of programs promoting wellness and disease management with more than 150 faith communities. She served as president of the Carolinas Health Ministry Partnership.

Jenny E. Holmes, MSN, RN
Faith Community Nurse

Jenny Holmes has 42 years of nursing experience, the past 18 years in faith community nursing.

She served in her faith community as a full-time parish nurse for 7 years before becoming the coordinator of an 80-member faith community nursing network. She has served as a Health Ministries Association Board member and in leadership roles in regional health ministry partnerships. Her community service includes American Heart Association BLS instructor and American Red Cross Volunteer heath reviewer.

Cassandra Howard, BSN, MAOM, RN-BC
Faith Community Nurse Consultant, CEO and Managing Partner of Community Outreach Resource and Education (CORE) Institute

Cassandra Howard is a faith community nurse with over 15 years' experience as a Lay Health Minister and a Westberg Institute for Faith Community Nursing curriculum educator. She has combined her strengths as an executive and managing businesswoman with her work in faith community nursing. She has developed community health improvement programs with community-based and nongovernmental organizations for the underserved demographics of the southern region primarily in Louisiana, Alabama, and Texas. Ms. Howard is a dynamic educator and mentor to over 300 faith community nurses and has provided leadership in the establishment of over 150 faith-based wellness partnerships. She achieved American Nurses Credentialing Center certification by portfolio in Faith Community Nursing in 2014.

Jennifer Knoulton, BSN, RN
Director of Nursing, Methodist Healthcare Ministries of South Texas, Inc., San Antonio, Texas

Jennifer Knoulton has 25 years of nursing experience: 10 years as a faith community nurse and currently as a director of nursing. The largest program under her leadership is the Wesley Nurse program, which partners with the Rio Texas conference of the United Methodist Church. The program has grown in the last 18 years to now include 80 full-time faith community nurses. This program provides faith community nursing to the underserved in a 74-county area of South Texas.

Deborah Ringen, MSN, PHN, BSN, RN-BC
Faith Community Nurse Adjunct Faculty Azusa Pacific University, Azusa California; Faith Community Nurse, Visiting Nurses of the Lower Valley, Centerbrook, Connecticut

Deborah Ringen has more than 30 years of nursing experience and earned her Master of Science in Nursing in Parish Nursing and Health Ministry from Azusa Pacific University. As a faith community nurse coordinator and educator, she has used her experience in home health nursing to help inform her practice. Deborah has completed one unit of Clinical Pastoral Education. She serves on the national United Church of Christ Faith Community Nurse Leadership Team. She achieved American Nurses Credentialing Center certification by portfolio in Faith Community Nursing in 2014.

Felicia D. Stewart, DNP, NP-C, RN-BC
Assistant Professor, School of Nursing, College of Health and Human Services, Indiana State University, Terre Haute, Indiana

Dr. Stewart has more than 20 years of nursing experience with the past 8 years as a board-certified family nurse practitioner. She was commissioned as a faith community nurse in 2012 while completing her Doctorate in Nursing Practice with her scholarly work focusing on the role of the advanced practice registered nurse in the faith community. She has served as a nonpaid faith community nurse, leader of health ministry, and at a free clinic for uninsured adults.

She is a member of the Indiana Conference United Methodist Church Faith Community Nursing/Health Ministry Committee. She achieved American Nurses Credentialing Center certification by portfolio as a faith community nurse in 2014.

Ruth Syre, MSN, RN-BC
Program Manager, Congregation and Community Health,
Centra, Lynchburg, Virginia

In a nursing career spanning more than forty years, over half of her career has been in community settings; most in leadership positions. She has served in her own congregation as a Faith Community Nurse since 1998. She has developed and implemented a system-wide health ministry program including Faith Community Nurses and Congregational Health Promoters, working with over 80 congregations. She is a Westberg Institute for Faith Community Nursing curriculum educator, and Vice Chair of the ANCC Content Expert Panel for Faith Community Nurse Certification. She achieved American Nurses Credentialing Center certification by portfolio as a faith community nurse in 2014.

Additional Contributors

Katora Campbell, DrPH, MSN, RN

Beverly Lunsford, PhD, CNS-BC, RN

Katia Reinert, PhD, MSN, RN, CRNP, RN-BC, PHCNS-BC

Angela Sheehan, MS, RN-BC, PMHNP-BC

Marsha Fowler, PhD, MDiv, MS, RN, FAAN

ANA Committee on Nursing Practice Standards

Danette Culver, MSN, APRN, ACNS-BC, CCRN, Co-Chair

Patricia Bowe, DNP, MS, RN, Co-Chair

Renee Gecsedi, MS, RN

Richard Henker, PhD, RN, CRNA, FAAN

Kirk Koyama, MSN, RN, CNS

Carla Lee, PhD, APRN-BC, CNAA, FAAN, FIBA

Tonette McAndrew, MPA, BSN, RN

Verna Sitzer, PhD, RN, CNS

Tom Blodgett, PhD, MSN, RN-BC, Alternate

Stacy McCall, MSN, RN, IBCLC, Alternate

ANA Staff

Carol J. Bickford, PhD, RN-BC, CPHIMS, FHIMSS, FAAN – Content editor

Joi Morris, BS, CAP-OM – Project coordinator

Lisa M. Myers, Esq. – Legal counsel

Liz Stokes, JD, RN – Ethics consultant

Erin E. Walpole, BA, PMP–Project editor

About the American Nurses Association

The American Nurses Association (ANA) is the only full-service professional organization representing the interests of the nation's 3.6 million registered nurses through its constituent member nurses' associations and its organizational affiliates. ANA advances the nursing profession by fostering high standards of nursing practice, promoting the rights of nurses in the workplace, projecting a positive and realistic view of nursing, and lobbying the Congress and regulatory agencies on healthcare issues affecting nurses and the public.

About the Health Ministries Association, Inc.

The Health Ministries Association, Inc. (HMA), a nonprofit membership organization, is the recognized professional membership organization for the nursing specialty of faith community nursing and promotes education, research utilization, and evidence-based practice. HMA is a support network for people of faith who promote whole-person health through faith groups in the communities they serve. By providing information, guidelines, and resources, HMA assists and encourages individuals, families, and communities as they develop whole-person health programs, utilize community resources, and educate others on the interdependent health of body, mind, and spirit. More details are available at www.hmassoc.org/.

About Nursebooks.org, The Publishing Program of ANA

Since the late 1990s ANA has partnered with other nursing organizations to establish a formal process for recognition of specialty areas of nursing practice. This includes the criteria for approving the specialty itself and the scope statement, and an acknowledgment by ANA of the standards of practice for that specialty. Because of the significant changes in the evolving nursing and healthcare environments, ANA's approval of specialty nursing scope statements and its acknowledgment of specialty standards of practice remain valid for five years, starting from the publication date of the documents.

Overview of the Content

The American Nurses Association recognizes faith community nursing as a nursing specialty. Faith community nursing acknowledges spiritual care as an essential component of a specialized body of nursing knowledge and competencies. A faith community nurse (hereafter, referred to as FCN; plural FCNs) provides care to individuals, families, groups, communities, and populations with emphasis on promoting whole-person health. As professional registered nurses, FCNs are guided in their decision-making and practice by the *Code of Ethics for Nurses With Interpretive Statements; Nursing Scope and Standards of Practice, Third Edition;* and *Guide to Nursing's Social Policy Statement: Understanding the Profession From Social Contract to Social Covenant.* These three documents form the foundation of practice for all registered nurses. Faith community nurses hold themselves accountable to the scope and standards of practice; state, commonwealth, or territory laws, statutes, and regulations related to nursing practice; and federal regulations.

Additional Content

For additional appreciation of the history and context related to *Faith Community Nursing Scope and Standards, Third Edition*, the reader will find additional useful content in the two appendices:

Appendix A. *Faith Community Nursing Scope and Standards, Second Edition*

Appendix B. Historic Milestones in Faith Community Nursing in the United States

Introduction

The American Nurses Association (ANA) published the first *Scope and Standards of Parish Nursing Practice* in 1998. As the practice of parish nursing evolved and included multiple faith traditions, the title of the specialty practice was changed to faith community nursing with the publication of *Faith Community Nursing: Scope and Standards of Practice* in 2005. Since the second revision in 2012, there have been dramatic changes in health care as well as the nursing profession. *Faith Community Nursing: Scope and Standards of Practice, Third Edition*, describes the current specialty practice of faith community nursing for the nursing profession, faith community nurses (FCNs), other healthcare providers, spiritual leaders, employers, insurers, healthcare consumers, families, and members of faith communities. The scope of practice statement presents the framework and context of faith community nursing practice and accompanies the standards of practice and professional performance and their associated competencies. The scope and standards included in this document define the responsibilities of the FCN and guide professional practice and performance.

The Standards of Practice encompass significant actions taken by registered nurses and form the foundation of the nurse's decision-making. The Standards of Professional Performance describe a competent level of behavior in the professional role, including activities related to ethics, culturally congruent practice, communication, collaboration, leadership, education, evidence-based practice and research, quality of practice, professional practice evaluation, resource utilization, and environmental health. "Registered nurses are accountable for their professional actions to themselves, their healthcare consumers, their peers, and ultimately to society" (ANA, 2015b, p. 5). In the application of standards to practice, the influence of context must be considered. "Whether a particular standard or competency applies depends on the circumstances" (ANA, 2015b, p. 6).

Function of the Scope of Practice Statement of Faith Community Nursing

The scope of practice statement describes the "who," "what," "where," "when," "why," and "how" of the practice of faith community nursing. The answers to these questions provide a comprehensive picture of the practice, its boundaries, and its membership. The scope of faith community nursing practice is specific to this specialty but builds on the scope of competent practice and professional performance expected of all registered nurses.

Function of the Standards of Faith Community Nursing Practice

Standards are "authoritative statements of the duties that all registered nurses, regardless of role, population, or specialty, are expected to perform competently" (ANA, 2015b, p. 3). Standards reflect the values and priorities of the profession and provide direction for professional nursing practice and a framework for evaluation of this practice. The ANA outlines six standards of professional nursing practice and 11 standards of professional performance. Competencies are included for each standard, which provide evidence of compliance with that particular standard. The standards included in this document define the responsibilities of the FCN and guide professional practice and performance.

Changes in health care and nursing practice may result in new context for this nursing specialty. The competencies related to each of the standards reflect current practice and provide details for application of the standards. The competencies listing is not meant to be exhaustive.

Application of the Scope and Standards

This third edition of the *Faith Community Nursing Scope and Standards of Practice* provides a valuable resource for FCNs to use in decision-making and when expanding, validating, or analyzing their professional practice. The document can be used to guide the development and evaluation of many aspects of faith community nursing practice including the following:

- Initial preparation and ongoing educational programs,
- Role description and performance evaluations,
- Policies and procedures,
- Quality improvement programs, and
- Processes for certification.

Summary

The scope and standards of practice for faith community nursing reflect the commitment of the Health Ministries Association (HMA) to partner with ANA to promote an understanding of faith community nursing as a specialized practice in the interprofessional practice of diverse faith communities. Due to the diversity of participating faith communities, it is important to identify inclusive terminology to describe the beliefs and practices related to varieties of faith traditions. Terms used in this document indicate an effort to include many faith traditions and not to promote any particular one. *Faith Community Nursing: Scope and Standards of Practice, Third Edition*, reflects current faith community nursing practice from a national perspective, the professional and ethical standards of the nursing profession, and the legal scope and standards of professional nursing practice. The standards are dynamic and subject to testing and change.

Scope of Faith Community Nursing Practice

Description of the Scope of Faith Community Nursing Practice

Faith community nursing is dynamic and evolves with changes in knowledge, the healthcare environment, and society. Faith community nurses (FCNs) include diploma, associate degree, baccalaureate-prepared registered nurses (RNs), graduate-level-prepared RNs, and advanced practice registered nurses (APRNs). The preferred minimum preparation for an RN or APRN entering the specialty of faith community nursing is a baccalaureate degree in nursing. The depth and breadth of an individual specialty nurse's scope of practice are determined by the nurse's education, experience, practice setting, role, and the specific population cared for by the nurse. Advanced practice RNs function within the full scope of their licensure incorporating the specialty focus in their practice.

Definition of Faith Community Nursing

Faith community nursing is a specialized practice of professional nursing that focuses on the intentional care of the spirit as well as the promotion of whole-person health and the prevention or minimization of illness within the context of a faith community and the wider community. An FCN is a registered professional nurse who is actively licensed in a given state and who serves as a member of the staff of a faith community. The FCN promotes health as wholeness of the faith community, its groups, families, and individual members through the practice of nursing as defined by that state's nurse practice act in the jurisdiction in which the FCN practices and the standards of practice set forth in this document.

The FCN promotes whole-person care across the life span using the skills of a professional nurse and provider of spiritual care (ANA, 2016). The FCN provides care during multiple encounters with healthcare consumers over extended periods of time, which may include stages of healthy growth and development as well as periods of change in functional level, illness, loss, and grief.

The FCN provides spiritual care in the faith community as well as in the broader community. The goals of an FCN are as follows:

- Protection, promotion, and optimization of health and abilities;

- Prevention of illness and injury;

- Facilitation of healing;

- Alleviation of suffering through the diagnosis and treatment of human responses; and

- Advocacy in the context of the values, beliefs, and practices of a faith community, such as a church, congregation, parish, synagogue, temple, mosque, or faith-based community agency.

Healthcare consumer is the term used by the ANA to define "a person, client, family, group, community, or population that is the focus of attention and to which the RN is providing services as sanctioned by the state regulatory bodies. This more global term is intended to reflect a proactive focus on health and wellness care, rather than a reactive perspective to disease and illness" (ANA, 2015b, p. 2). In narratives within the specialty of faith community nursing, other terms such as parishioner, congregant, or faith community member may also be included as descriptive terms. The term healthcare consumer may refer to the faith community or broader community as a whole or to groups, families, and individuals in the faith community.

The Specialty of Faith Community Nursing

The FCN uses the nursing process to assess and address the spiritual, physical, mental, and social health of the healthcare consumer. With an intentional focus on spiritual health, the FCN primarily uses evidence-based practice interventions such as health education, counseling, prayer, presence, active listening, advocacy, referrals, and a wide variety of other resources available to the faith community. The FCN may also provide education and supervision to volunteers from the faith community. As an actively licensed RN, the FCN provides nursing care based on standards and professional experience, legal expectations, and education. The FCN focuses on the assets and needs as defined by both the faith community and the healthcare consumer population. The FCN collaborates with interprofessional teams in a variety of settings including healthcare systems, integrative health, mental health, social work, long-term care, as well as denominations, faith-based organizations and other community agencies to enhance nursing care and promote quality outcomes.

Faith community nurses continue to advocate for public policy that addresses health disparities and promotes health and wellness (HMA/ANA, 2012, p. 10). In faith community settings, the FCN advocates for appropriate levels of care and access to care for vulnerable populations. Faith community nurses advocate for healthcare consumers by initiating referrals for community services, promoting health literacy, and providing health education to empower individuals to manage their health concerns.

Distinguishing Tenets of Faith Community Nursing

The specialty practice of faith community nursing includes the application of nursing science and practice to individuals of all ages within a faith community setting and the surrounding community. The differentiating factor from general nursing practice is the specific attention that is given to the intentional care of the spirit. The FCN delivers care that promotes whole-person-centered well-being, establishes a therapeutic relationship that acknowledges caring as a sacred practice, and focuses on the relationship between faith and health.

A person's faith beliefs, rituals, spiritual practices, and health views are a central focus in relationships formed by FCNs to provide nursing and spiritual care.

The FCN engages in intentional conversations with persons about how these factors interplay with their health and well-being. "Use of compassionate listening and reflective open dialogue enables individuals to express their understanding of how healing happens for them and how they can be supported" (HMA, 2017). The interventions of active listening, prayer, and therapeutic touch are intentionally incorporated into the FCN's caring presence. This specialty practice holds that all persons are sacred and must be treated with dignity and respect. The foundations of the specialty practice are in accordance with the ANA's statements about nursing and the essence of the practice.

Essential to the practice of faith community nursing is a caring relationship that promotes trust and the understanding of health as a dynamic process that embodies the spiritual, physical, mental, and social dimensions of the person. Faith community nursing practice is influenced by the theoretical principles of effective caring to promote health and individual or family growth. Every human experience has mind–body–spirit components. Attention to identified human responses is accomplished by practicing an approach to health promotion and wholeness that recognizes that the mind, body, and spirit are intertwined. Particular emphasis is placed on the spiritual component, particularly as it relates to whole-person health.

Foundations of Practice

The practice of faith community nursing remains based on the assumptions that

- Health and illness are human experiences;
- Health is the integration of the spiritual, physical, psychological, and social aspects of the person promoting a sense of harmony with self, others, the environment, and a higher power;
- Health may be experienced in the presence of disease or injury;
- The presence of illness does not preclude health nor does optimal health preclude illness; and
- Healing is the process of integrating the body, mind, and spirit to create wholeness, health, and a sense of well-being, even when the healthcare consumer's illness is not cured (HMA/ANA, 2012, p. 8).

This specialized practice is a continually evolving practice requiring integration of new knowledge and awareness of ever-changing resources to achieve desired outcomes. Faith community nurses appraise nursing practice standards, position statements, and evidence-based publications from peer-reviewed professional journals for optimal application in their practice.

The core values of faith community nursing embrace four major concepts that are adapted from a faith community nursing curriculum [International Parish Nurse Resource Center (IPNRC), 2014, p. 5]:

- Spiritual formation: an ongoing, essential component of practice that includes both self-care and hospitality, through opening the heart to self and others as well as an intentional process of fostering spiritual growth;
- Professionalism: practicing under the *Faith Community Nursing: Scope and Standards of Practice* and the ANA *Code of Ethics*;
- Whole-person health: an understanding of health as a dynamic process that embodies the spiritual, physical, mental, and social dimensions of the person; and
- Community: fostering new and creative responses to health and wellness in partnership with other community health resources.

Settings

Faith community nurse practice is nursing care that focuses on intentional care of the spirit and is practiced within the context of a faith community. A community of faith may be composed of people of all ages. The FCN provides nursing care to pediatric, adolescent, adult, and geriatric members of the faith community who represent a diverse range of cognitive and functional abilities. An individual, family, group, or the faith community as a whole may experience or desire a change in their level of spiritual, physical, mental, social, or environmental well-being or desire to maintain their current level of well-being. The FCN collaborates with them to develop a plan of care that incorporates communal and individual spiritual beliefs and practices.

The needs and desires of individual members of the faith community provide direction for the FCN interaction and often require that the FCN visit members in a hospital or hospice, private home, or residential facility or accompany healthcare consumers as they navigate health services within the community and beyond. During these encounters, the FCN integrates faith and health and provides a supportive, healing presence for the healthcare consumer, caregiver, and others.

The settings for faith community nursing continue to expand as the needs of populations grow and change. While the traditional setting is often a community of faith—a church or congregation, a synagogue, temple, or mosque— nontraditional settings may also include faith-based health clinics, day shelters, food pantries, senior centers, long-term care facilities, and other community settings. Faith-based community sites for underserved populations that provide food, housing, and resources may also incorporate FCNs for chronic disease management, screenings, health education, and ongoing whole-person care (Balint & George, 2015). Faith community nurses have reached out to nursing colleagues in schools of nursing to provide lectures on spirituality and health and serve as clinical preceptors for community health nursing students. Faith community nurses are also partnering with healthcare and community organizations to provide educational presentations to nursing colleagues in transitional care, home health, and hospice settings.

Faith community nurses practice in urban and rural settings and have the opportunity to impact health care in a proactive manner and link individuals and families to resources within their faith community and the surrounding community. Each setting and each community are unique. Health issues in these communities may include concentrations of several populations who experience poor health, such as individuals with substance abuse problems, victims of violence, individuals with chronic and persistent mental illness, the disabled, and people living with HIV. Other issues needing attention may include access to health resources and care; transportation; health literacy; safety and environmental concerns; effective emergency medical system (EMS) resources; access to mental health care; social isolation; and financial concerns. Presenting an additional challenge, approximately one in five Americans—nearly 60 million people—lives in a rural area (U.S. Census, 2016). For many, medical care is miles away, and a fully equipped hospital still farther (Robert Wood Johnson, 2010). This results in the sobering fact that the farther patients need to travel for care, the more likely they are to put off medical appointments or not seek care (Modern Health Care, 2014). Identification of both the assets and needs of the community will guide the activities of the FCN as various issues are addressed. The FCN identifies resources within the faith community and local and regional partners to optimize health care and employ creative avenues to meet the needs of the population served.

The size, concerns, assets, and expectations of the faith community will help define and guide the development of the FCN's expected role. As a staff member, the paid or unpaid FCN is most often supported and guided by a committee of faith community leaders and assisted by lay volunteers. With education and supervision provided by the FCN, these volunteers may assume tasks that family members would do for each other if they were available. Faith community nurses may be managers of health and wellness programs with responsibilities for budget preparation and oversight, strategic planning, coordination with other initiatives of the faith community and/or healthcare systems, and supervision and performance evaluation of volunteers.

Evolution of Faith Community Nursing

Nursing has its historical foundation deeply rooted in faith and health, as well as in the ancient and recent traditions of many religions. Faith traditions established public health practices, including care of persons with infectious diseases. These communities also included visiting the sick and caring for infants and the elderly as religious duty. This sense of duty to care for a community's members expanded to include "care for the stranger" and was the basis for early *diakonas*—houses for strangers—which became the first charity hospitals.

The faith and health link evolved over time and has been influenced by cultural, political, social, and economic events. Religious groups founded hospitals to provide care to vulnerable populations, such as the poor, immigrant, and homeless. In the 12th, 13th, and 14th centuries, religious orders provided care for persons with physical and mental illnesses. During the 16th century, more than 100 female religious orders were founded specifically to provide care to the sick, wounded, and mentally ill. These were precursors to nursing practice.

In the late 1800s, churches began to reclaim their role in healing. Diaconal ministries that developed in Europe migrated to the United States, and immigrant churches imported the work of deaconesses and other religious orders to provide health care to those in their communities. These religious affiliations were instrumental in developing schools of nursing during the 20th century. Florence Nightingale, trained through the Deaconess Institution in

Kaiserswerth, Germany, felt called to the service of the sick. In addition to her nursing education, she was a theological scholar and writer. Her religious philosophy and belief in a higher power were the foundations for her work to promote nursing as a trained profession, establish a public healthcare system that included health promotion and preventive medicine, and advocate for health issues as a social activist. The rich history of nursing's evolution is exquisitely collected in *Nursing, The Finest Art: An Illustrated History* (Donahue, 1996).

In the late 1950s, Halbert Dunn, a physician, developed a public health concept that he called high-level wellness. His writings were a catalyst for wellness centers that began in the 1970s (Dunn, 1959). A growing public interest in complementary and alternative medicine influenced Western conventional medical care to incorporate aspects of these models into integrated care. This growing interest and focus on health promotion and wellness influenced the development of faith community nursing.

In 1973, Rev. Dr. Granger Westberg, in conjunction with W.K. Kellogg Foundation and the Department of Preventive Medicine and Community Health of the University of Illinois College of Medicine, began medical clinics in neighborhood churches located in marginalized communities, which he termed Wholistic Health Centers. The intent was to bring about whole-person health care in faith settings by having spiritually oriented doctors, nurses, social workers, and clergy working together. The nurses in these "wholistic health centers" were referred to as "parish nurses." The word "wholistic" has been associated with the movement championed by Granger Westberg. It has been a defining descriptor that served to identify the focus of nursing care as the specialty of faith community nursing developed. The current ANA definition of "holistic care" encompasses all the characteristics embodied in whole-person health care provided by FCNs (see glossary). Both terms may be used in publications. The focus of faith community nursing care, whole-person health and wellness, remains constant.

In 1986, the Parish Nurse Resource Center was created through the sponsorship of Lutheran General Health System (now Advocate Health Care) in Chicago. The center provided a national focal point for the development of parish nursing through its educational resources. With the expansion of the practice to other countries, the name was changed in 2001 to the International Parish Nurse Resource Center (IPNRC). The IPNRC was relocated in 2002 to St. Louis under the management of the Deaconess Foundation until 2011, when it was moved to the Church Health Center in Memphis. In 2016, the name of the center was changed to the Westberg Institute for Faith Community Nursing.

In 1989, a 3-year Kellogg Foundation grant supported the development of the HMA. The HMA was incorporated as a nonprofit membership organization in Iowa to provide communication and networking among FCNs.

In 1990, HMA received a grant from the Kellogg Foundation through the Northwest Aging Association in Iowa to establish staff and begin programming. The same year, HMA received a 3-year grant from Wheat Ridge Foundation to begin 70 health ministry programs in faith communities. The organization logo was adopted and chapter development authorized at the first Annual HMA Meeting and Conference in Northbrook, Chicago, in 1991.

During the 1990s, education for faith community nursing was becoming formalized. In 1991, the first basic preparation continuing education (CE) course, called the Wisconsin model, was taught by Rosemarie Matheus through Concordia University and later at Marquette University. The Parish Nurse Resource Center developed standardized CE curricula for parish nurses, educators, and coordinators. This paved the way for other university schools of nursing to offer the Parish Nurse Resource Center's curriculum as CE. Georgetown University and Marquette University also offered parish nursing preparatory courses as nonmatriculated undergraduate credit courses. From 2001 to 2009, Duke University offered a master's degree in Health and Nursing Ministries, which was a joint initiative of the School of Nursing and Duke Divinity School. The IPNRC offers an annual CE conference, The Westberg Symposium, and the HMA hosts an annual meeting and CE conference.

In the 1990s and early 2000s, healthcare systems received local, regional, and/or national foundation grants to develop outreach programs with partnering faith communities for health promotion and disease prevention. The primary operational model consisted of a coordinator, who was a paid employee of the healthcare system, with paid and/or unpaid FCNs located in faith communities. These grants were usually funded as a 3-year cycle and many programs were not sustained after the grant cycle ended. In contrast, some of the early programs in several regions of the country continue today and achieve significant health outcomes through case-finding, referral, and improved access to care.

In 1997, the HMA's formal request to the ANA was approved and ANA recognized parish nursing as a professional nursing specialty. In 1998, ANA accepted and published HMA's *Scope and Standards of Parish Nursing Practice.* In 2005, revision of the text resulted in a title change to *Faith Community Nursing: Scope and Standards of Practice* to be inclusive of nurses in all faith traditions. In 2010, HMA held its first National Summit at Burlingame, California. A white paper, *Now More Than Ever*, was published through grant support of the Health and Human Services Office on Women's Health, Washington, DC. The HMA established two awards for excellence: The Wilkerson-Droege Award in honor of Sister June Wilkerson and Reverend Thomas Droege was first awarded in 2002, and the Westberg Faith Community Nursing Leadership Award was first awarded in 2012.

In 2012, *Faith Community Nursing: Scope and Standards of Practice, Second Edition*, was revised by HMA and published by ANA. The standards of faith community nursing practice and professional practice were incorporated into curricula, position descriptions, and performance evaluation processes. This intentional focus on professional nursing practice provided the foundational work for advancement of the specialty.

Since 2007, the HMA has been working with the American Nurses Credentialing Center (ANCC) to develop certification in faith community nursing. This work culminated in 2014 with ANCC offering Certification by Portfolio in Faith Community Nursing. In 2015, HMA established the Faith Community Nursing Society to recognize nurses who have achieved certification by portfolio in faith community nursing. The HMA continues to provide education and practice support for FCNs and others in healing ministries through their national conference, publications, and membership services. In March 2017, HMA joined ANA as an Organizational Affiliate. Historical milestones of faith community nursing in the United States are summarized in Appendix B.

The "what" and "how" of nursing includes use of evidence-based practice, care coordination, and the ethical manner in which the nurse practices (ANA, 2015b, pp. 7–9). There has been significant evolution and growth in faith community nursing over time while remaining grounded in whole-person care. Early literature identified seven roles as the original "functions" or "roles" of the FCN: integrator of faith and health, personal health counselor, health educator, health advocate, referral agent, coordinator of volunteers, and developer of support groups (Hickman, 2006; Westberg & McNamara, 1990). Smucker (2008) describes the transition to the FCN role as "being and doing." Her textbook also describes a model for Jewish congregational nursing. More recently, these traditional roles have been analyzed and attributes of FCNs collected in descriptive studies continue to be reported (Solari-Twadell & Hackbarth, 2010). When implementing the nursing process, FCNs use a whole-person-centered approach in their dynamic processes of assessment, diagnosis, identification of outcomes, planning, implementation, and evaluation. The "how" and "what" of an FCN's practice are determined by the assets and needs of the faith community. Nurse-led programs within faith communities continue to grow and evolve. Faith community nurses impact the health and wellness of individuals, families, communities, and populations. The common expectation across faith traditions is that the professional RN functioning as an FCN possesses a depth of understanding of the faith community's traditions, as well as competence as an RN.

Focus on Spiritual Care

Nurses have long observed that when illness or brokenness occurs, health-care consumers, whether individually or with family or friends, often turn to their source of spiritual strength for reassurance, support and healing. *Nursing: Scope and Standards of Practice, Third Edition* (ANA, 2015b), reaffirms that spiritual care is integral in all nursing practice. In the 2008 revision of the *Essentials of Baccalaureate Education for Professional Nursing Practice*, the presence of spiritual care and spiritual assessment in nursing curriculum was expanded to ensure that the basic education programs prepared nurses to conduct spiritual assessments and provide spiritual care. The nursing specialty of faith community nursing emphasizes spiritual care or intentional care of the spirit as an essential domain requiring additional education and skill beyond spiritual care provided in the general practice of an RN.

The FCN uses the nursing process for assessment, diagnosis, planning, implementation, and evaluation of nursing care for individuals, families, communities, and populations. Diagnosis terminology is applied across the general nursing profession through the use of standardized terminology such as in the NANDA International, Inc., comprehensive list of nursing diagnoses, including diagnoses on spiritual, physical, and emotional health. Nursing diagnoses related to spirituality include Spiritual Distress, Risk for Spiritual Distress, and Readiness for Enhanced Spiritual Well-being. Other nursing diagnoses accepted by NANDA International, Inc. that are related specifically to spirituality include Powerlessness, Hopelessness, Ineffective Coping, and Complicated Grieving (NANDA, 2012).

Faith community nurses may also use nursing classification systems. The Facilitation Center for Nursing Classification and Clinical Effectiveness groupings of Nursing Interventions Classifications and Nursing Outcomes Classifications represent common standardized systems for nursing interventions and evaluating the effects of the interventions (i.e., outcomes) used across nursing, including faith community nursing. Examples applicable to faith community nursing's focus on spiritual care giving include hope instillation, spiritual support, religious ritual enhancement, and spiritual growth.

The Omaha System is a standardized language developed for home, public health, and school health (Martin & Monsen, 2016). It is intended for use across the continuum of care for individuals, families, and communities who represent all ages, geographic locations, medical diagnoses, socioeconomic ranges, spiritual beliefs, ethnicity, and cultural values. Four domains—environmental, psychosocial, physiological, and health-related behaviors—provide the structure for three relational, reliable, and valid components designed to be used together:

- Problem Classification Scheme (client assessment)
- Intervention Scheme (care plans and services)
- Problem Rating Scale for Outcomes (client change/evaluation)

Examples of problems included in the psychosocial domain include the following:

- Role change
- Interpersonal relationship
- Spirituality
- Grief
- Mental health
- Sexuality
- Caretaking/parenting
- Abuse

The Clinical Care Classification System (CCC), formerly Home Health Care Classification System, developed by Dr. Virginia Saba, offers an approach for documenting nursing diagnoses, interventions, and outcomes of patient care in an electronic health record (EHR) system. The CCC lists use 21 standardized coded concepts to record nursing diagnoses, interventions, and outcomes. Five of these concepts closely correlate to faith community nursing: coping, health behavioral, role (relationship), self-concept, and life cycle (Saba, 2017).

Concept	Examples of Elements
Coping	Decisional conflict
	Posttrauma response
	Spiritual state alteration grieving
Health behavioral	Health maintenance alteration
	Health-seeking behavior
Role (relationship)	Parental role conflict
	Caregiver role strain
	Social isolation
Self-concept	Hopelessness
	Body image disturbance
	Situational self-esteem disturbance
Life cycle	Pregnancy risk
	Perinatal risk
	Growth and development alteration

Faith community nurses draw on professional skills that integrate spiritual care and nursing care, as well as the resources of individuals and groups both within and beyond the faith community, to provide whole-person care. Faith community nurses may also incorporate wellness diagnoses for health promotion that accentuate strengths and assets rather than illness or deficits and incorporate a person's positive aspects of life and health into their nursing care (Leddy, 2006; Stolte, 1996). Stolte cites several examples of wellness nursing diagnoses related to spirituality:

- Progressive religious faith,
- Maintaining strong spiritual foundation,
- Maintaining hope and trust,
- Progressive ability to forgive self and/or others,
- Continued belief in meaning and purpose of life, and
- At peace with self and/or health status.

Treatment may or may not cure an affliction. However, it is still possible for a person to experience healing through care of the spirit even if a cure—physical restoration—does not occur. A person may be dying of cancer, but if a broken relationship between family members has been reconciled or the person is at peace with the circumstances, this may be considered healing. This broader viewpoint of healing is embraced by FCNs.

Assault, betrayal, accident, and death of a member of the community are examples of situations that can affect an entire faith community. Members of all ages may manifest anger, grief, depression, anxiety, fear, and spiritual or physical pain in varying degrees. An FCN's response to such an event is complex. Beyond identifying and meeting the needs of individuals and families, the FCN treats the whole faith community as a healthcare consumer. Assessment focuses on identifying the educational and supportive needs of the whole faith community. Interventions occur at three different levels: community, family or group, and individual.

The FCN continues to address a variety of issues that threaten the health and wellbeing of persons in the faith community, including the following:

- Individuals or families may lack food, shelter, transportation, income, or health care;

- Victims of violence, abuse, or exploitation in a variety of settings, including domestic settings, may seek solace or sanctuary;

- Adult children of aging parents may seek guidance in talking with or determining the appropriate living situation for a parent, and ongoing assistance from the faith community; and

- Victims of natural disasters and other life-altering emergencies may require various forms of assistance (HMA/ANA, 2012, p. 9).

Some healthcare consumers will require support of basic needs so they have the time and space to reflect on spiritual issues; for others, spiritual care will be the direct response. The form of spiritual care will depend on the beliefs and practices of the faith community; the desire of the faith community, the group, or the individual; the skills of the FCN; and the collaboration of other staff members and volunteers.

Ethics in Faith Community Nursing

The *Code of Ethics for Nurses with Interpretive Statements* (ANA, 2015a) is foundational to nursing practice and serves as a guide to the art and science of nursing. The values in the Code apply to nurses in all roles, forms of practice, and settings. "The nine provisions in the Code are an expression of the values, virtues, and obligations that shape, guide, and inform nursing as a profession" (ANA, 2015a, p. vii). The provisions reflect three relationships: "nurse-to-patient," "nurse-to-profession," and "nurse-to-society." The interpretive statements of each provision provide guidance for ethical nursing practice and behavior. Note: within the *Code of Ethics for Nurses With Interpretive Statements* (ANA, 2015a), the contributors recognize and use the historic, more commonly used term, *patient*, as representative of all consumers of health care or individuals and groups of clients who are receiving care.

Faith community nurses promote whole-person health with intentional inclusion of religious or spiritual well-being and supportive care. Ethical healthcare issues require nonjudgmental therapeutic nurse–patient relationships. Faith community nurses may

- Guide conversations about care decisions arising at the intersection of faith beliefs and medically prescribed care;

- Serve as a person's healthcare advocate by accompanying them to medical appointments, defining medical terms, and interpreting medical therapies that are not understood;

- Promote development of persons' self-advocacy skills in order to empower them to make informed decisions related to their health and wellness; and

- Guide discussions on advance care planning, minimize unwarranted or unnecessary medical treatment, and provide compassionate end-of-life care.

Moral Distress

A nurse has a primary commitment to the recipients of nursing and healthcare services. Faith community nurses use the nursing process, the healthcare consumer's perspective, and the spiritual beliefs of a faith community as the basis for assessing a person's experience. Nurses assure that interventions are appropriate to optimize the health and well-being of those receiving care.

Andrew Jameton defined "moral distress" as a phenomenon in which one knows the right action to take but is constrained from taking it (Jameton, 1984). Moral distress occurs when the internal environment of nurses—their values and perceived obligations—are incompatible with the needs and prevailing views of the external work environment (Corley, 2002). The *Code of Ethics for Nurses* defines moral distress as the "condition of knowing the morally right thing to do, but institutional, procedural, or social constraints make doing the right thing nearly impossible. This condition threatens core values and moral integrity" (ANA, 2015a, p. 44).

In the context of faith community nursing, the tenets, beliefs, and practices of a faith group add another layer to the complexity of moral healthcare decision-making. Potential conflict may arise when there are differences between the faith community's religious view, the nurse's personal moral view, and the values and free will of the healthcare consumer. These decisional conflicts may arise in circumstances across the life span, treatment participation, socioeconomic challenges, and lifestyle choices.

The *Code of Ethics* provision 1 states that the nurse "practices with compassion and respect for the inherent dignity, worth, and unique attributes of every person" (ANA, 2015a, p. 1). Faith community nurses have a moral obligation to seek guidance when the rights of the individual person, public health doctrines, and religious views are in conflict. As moral agents, FCNs have a responsibility to express moral perspectives and provide information and resources that facilitate discernment and decision-making by the patient and family. "When nurses care for those whose health condition, attributes, lifestyle, or situations are stigmatized, or encounter a conflict with their personal beliefs, nurses must render compassionate, respectful, and competent care" (ANA, 2015a, p. 20). Faith community nurses, as moral agents and professional nurses, advocate for the best interests of patients, families, or communities.

Moral Resilience

Developing moral resilience provides the FCN with support during these circumstances.

> "Moral resilience represents the cultivation of skills and practices that support clinicians in deepening their connection and commitment to their primary intentions, recognizing their sense of moral responsibility, and effectively navigating ethically complex, ambiguous, or conflicting situations." (Rushton, Schoonover-Shoffner, & Kennedy, 2017)

Faith community nurses approach ethical and moral conflicts intentionally respecting the perspective of the individual and colleagues while extending same respect to self. The nursing process may guide the nurse in these challenging circumstances. Other examples of frameworks for ethical decision-making include a four-box method, which includes clinical indications, patient preferences, quality of life, and contextual features (Jonsen, Siegler, & Winslade, 2006) and a model incorporating four principles of biomedical ethics—autonomy, beneficence, nonmaleficence, and justice (Beauchamp & Childress, 2009).

Exemplars

The following exemplars from faith community nursing practice illustrate the nine provisions of the *Code of Ethics for Nurses With Interpretive Statements* (ANA, 2015a):

Provision 1
The nurse practices with compassion and respect for the inherent dignity, worth, and unique attributes of every person.

Faith communities participate in the resettlement and support of refugees from many parts of the world. The FCN works in a large faith community that hosts two different groups of refugees. When assisting a young woman of one refugee community, the FCN identifies symptoms that suggest a significant medical problem. In their initial discussion about a referral to a medical provider, the woman hesitates to agree with completing the referral. She defers until another meeting.

The FCN asks the woman to explain how she will approach this decision and learns that the impact of her decision is considered by the entire family and its interdependence that guides a collective approach to decision-making in this culture's views of health and healing. The FCN uses appreciative inquiry to learn about this culture's folk healing practices and beliefs. The FCN learns how prayer, visions, dreams or divination influence care and the interconnections of the spiritual and natural world in response to illness and its treatment. This culture's ancestral system weaves illness and cause together with the collective wisdom of family members (living and dead).

The FCN agrees to meet with the woman after she has shared the nurse's assessment and concern with her family. At the woman's request, the FCN provides written information about the symptoms and their potential cause, traditional medical treatment options, and outcomes. The woman shares this information with her family and also with the elders of their community. The following week, the woman invites the FCN to meet with her family to learn from them about their views on her health and the folk practices they suggest. In this gathering, the FCN portrays her role as an invited guest and listens attentively to questions from family members and their plans for the woman's treatment. The FCN informs the family that she will accompany the woman to medical appointments to assure that the healthcare providers are aware of these cultural views and preferences. The eldest family member gives permission for the appointment to be made.

The FCN accompanies the woman to the medical appointment and "creates the bridge between professional and folk health care systems" as described by Leininger and McFarland (2002). The FCN encourages the woman to inform the medical provider of the influence of the extended family in decision-making and the role of the culture's folk practices important in achieving health. With the advocacy of the FCN, the woman's diagnostic and treatment phases are a facilitated approach that preserves, accommodates, and restructures aspects of the culture's folk practices and incorporates them in the western approaches to care.

Provision 2
The nurse's primary commitment is to the patient, whether an individual, family, group, community, or population.

Family caregivers are often challenged to provide care of a loved one (patient/individual) living at a distance to include patient safety, managing activities of daily living, and recognizing changes in the patient's condition warranting further medical intervention. In these instances, the FCN is uniquely positioned to provide support for the person and family by knowledge of resources available in the faith community as well as the community at large to promote quality of life for both.

Over time, the FCN developed a trusting relationship with an elderly couple whose daughter lived out of state. When the daughter realized the needs of her parents were becoming more than she could provide from a distance, she contacted the FCN acknowledging the relationship developed with her parents. At the request of the daughter and with the permission of her parents, the FCN made an initial home assessment. The elderly couple wanted to remain in their home even if additional care was necessary at a future time. The FCN planned to make an observational home visit to the couple weekly and communicate findings to the daughter. Several months later, the FCN observed an increasing need for additional levels of in-home assistance to assure safety.

The FCN informed the daughter and arranged to meet with her during her next visit to her parents. They discussed the couple's need for increased assistance with activities of daily living. The FCN provided the daughter with information on area home care agencies and the daughter arranged for supportive home care. The FCN continued her weekly home visits and served as a facilitator for the elderly couple and the daughter's interactions with care attendants. The daughter was able to have assurance that care was being provided to her parents, continue working, enjoy quality visits with her parents, and honor the request of her parents to remain in their home for as long as possible. The FCN's ongoing assessment during home visits and communication and support to the daughter resulted in a safe environment and quality of life for the elderly couple.

Provision 3
The nurse promotes, advocates for, and protects the rights, health, and safety of the patient.
The FCN protects the rights, health, and safety of the patient by ensuring confidentiality and by ensuring policy and procedure is in place to promote a culture of safety and quality of care. Confidentiality in faith community nursing practice extends beyond the individual patient to the family and others involved in a particular circumstance.

Faith community nursing practice requires diligence in maintaining confidentiality. In one encounter, the faith leader asks the FCN for information regarding a particular faith community member's health to plan spiritual visits and support. The FCN replies that the person has not given permission to share the information and the FCN has an obligation to protect the person's health information.

Faith community members acquainted with another faith community member ask the FCN questions about the person's health during a recent illness and hospitalization. They are planning to add the person's name to the weekly prayer list in which members pray for those who are ill or in crisis. The FCN educates these faith community members about protection of personal health information, confidentiality standards, and the necessity of obtaining consent of a person to include their name or information on a prayer list. The FCN writes an addendum to the procedure for creating the weekly prayer list to include instructions about maintaining confidentiality and not disclosing personal health information without consent.

The FCN informs the faith leader and community members of the ethical and legal requirements for protection of personal health information and ethical provisions and standards essential to nurse–patient confidentiality. Patient/family consent is required to disclose any information or circumstances to anyone including healthcare providers, clergy, or social service agencies. The FCN holds all knowledge of patient/family circumstances in confidence until consent is obtained.

Provision 4
The nurse has authority, accountability, and responsibility for nursing practice, makes decisions, and takes action consistent with the obligation to promote health and to provide optimum care.

The FCN is asked by the congregational leader to visit a church member recently hospitalized with heart failure. Upon receiving permission from the faith community member, a home visit is made to an elderly couple, the husband having been discharged two days prior. The nurse completed an assessment, including physical assessment, medication understanding and compliance, nutritional understanding and compliance, awareness of warning signs and appropriate responses, and follow-up plans. In addition, a spiritual assessment was conducted, particularly for indications of spiritual distress. Following assessment, the nurse, in conjunction with the couple, established a plan of care, including weekly visitation to continue assessment, review of medication and dietary compliance, support, and encouragement. The FCN, upon request, offers a prayer for health and peace for the couple.

On subsequent visits over the next 2 weeks, the nurse assessed that medications were being taken consistently, but the couple was eating foods containing large amounts of salt, which were long-standing behaviors. When questioned, the couple stated they were not going to change their eating habits. The recommended dietary changes were distasteful to them. The husband exhibited increased ankle edema and some shortness of breath. The FCN realizes that this lack of compliance may lead to impaired health, repeated hospitalizations, and diminished quality and quantity of life. This moral conflict impedes the ability of the FCN to promote optimum health. This may contribute to spiritual distress for the FCN, as this impacts the concept of caring for the gift of life. However, the FCN also recognizes the principles of autonomy, beneficence, and nonmaleficence.

The FCN shares concerns with the couple of the possible consequences of noncompliance with dietary guidelines. The couple verbalizes understanding and clearly articulates the comfort of familiar food as a component of quality of life for them. They agree to continued visitation and are open to continued discussion of possible dietary alterations. They verbalize appreciation of the spiritual support from the FCN and agree to have the faith community leader informed of their status.

The FCN recognizes that the personal choices the couple has made are in conflict with the FCN's personal values and knowledge of the potential for resulting negative impact. This provides an opportunity for the FCN to self-examine values and teaching effectiveness. While responsible for nursing practice, the FCN must remain respectful of others' right to make choices regarding their own health care.

Provision 5
The nurse owes the same duties to self as to others, including the responsibility to promote health and safety, preserve wholeness of character and integrity, maintain competence, and continue personal and professional growth.

During worship, a couple asked the FCN to pray for their young son recently diagnosed with autism. The parents were overwhelmed by this information at a recent visit with their pediatrician. The FCN obtained the parents' permission to share this medical information with the pastor. Prior to meeting with the pastor to discuss support for this family, the FCN reviewed encounter records and noted that this was the fourth family she met with in the two previous months who were experiencing this life circumstance. Each of these families turned to their faith community for understanding, acceptance, and support as they sought to respond emotionally and spiritually to their child's needs.

The FCN and pastor discussed how the faith community could welcome these families and have them feel included in community life. Both the FCN and pastor identified a personal need for gaining a better understanding of autism and how to provide support. They discussed maintaining the confidentiality of those families that did not want information shared while other parents shared information with friends and teachers. Teachers were asking for information so they could be more supportive to these parents.

The FCN contacted the state's autism society and learned of a workshop for faith communities to help families of children and adults with autism. The pastor and FCN attended the conference and obtained educational materials on autism. The FCN contacted a pediatric nursing colleague to gain additional medical knowledge about autism. The FCN met with a legal counselor to learn about state obligations for services and the rights of adults with autism including housing, employment training, and day services.

The FCN's educational sessions provided Information on behavior patterns across the autism spectrum, emphasis on early screening and diagnosis, local resources, and a narrative shared by one family of their personal experiences.

Additional sessions were provided for staff and teachers focusing on inclusion of children with special needs. The FCN joined the autism society network to receive ongoing information. The FCN and pastor continued to meet with parents who sought the support of their faith community in order to be responsive to changing needs of their children. Maintaining competence is an ongoing process that broadens the FCN's self-understanding and advances excellence in providing care.

Provision 6
The nurse, through individual and collective effort, establishes, maintains, and improves the ethical environment of the work setting and conditions of employment that are conducive to safe, quality health care.

Faith community nurses have a unique role in working with other professionals who are generally not healthcare providers and therefore may have limited or no understanding of HIPAA and other rules/laws which guide professional nursing/FCN practice.

An FCN works in a faith community that has engaged in ministry with a local domestic violence shelter to support the women and children seeking services. The FCN envisions using nursing assessment, varied educational and clinical experience, resource knowledge, and advocacy skills to work with this local ministry effort. The congregational team is excited to have the FCN on-board and has ideas for the nurse's work. The associate faith community leader would like the FCN to participate in weekly round-table staff discussions of specific issues concerning the clients. The FCN is excited about the depth of engagement and commitment to these women and children but recognizes that there is an expectation that the FCN share protected health information (PHI) with the group.

Healthcare providers, including professional nurses, are bound by the Health Insurance Portability and Accountability Act of 1996 (HIPAA). The HIPAA includes the Privacy Rule, which limits the use of PHI in order to minimize the chances of inappropriate use. Professional nurses are also bound by state boards of nursing, which serve to protect patients' and their rights. Professional nurses also follow the provisions of the Nursing Code of Ethics, which emphasize the obligation of professional nurses to protect patients, including their dignity and privacy, and inform what the FCN can share.

The FCN reports that discussion will be limited to general knowledge only of needs and strengths without discussing specific clients. The other faith community members respond with anger and comments regarding the FCN's lack of compassion, and the staff's perception of the nurse being an impediment to helping the women in the shelter. The associate faith community leader appreciates the FCN professional skills but fails to understand how the FCN can contribute meaningful work without giving specific information during the weekly group meetings. The associate leader asks the FCN to reconsider sharing specific client information.

The FCN cites professional nursing standards and states she cannot compromise in this situation. The FCN explains to the associate leader that relaying health information about a particular person at the shelter or one receiving treatment for a mental health issue may have a potentially harmful effect. With this new knowledge and understanding of how HIPAA applies to the FCN practice, the associate faith community leader now supports the FCN and advocates confidentiality with the mission group and the congregation. The FCN also uses this as an opportunity to educate the group on their own health information privacy rights.

Provision 7
The nurse, in all roles and settings, advances the profession through research and scholarly inquiry, professional standards development, and the generation of both nursing and health policy.

Faith community nurses may conduct research or explore the published literature to determine whether the current evidence necessitates a change in practice. These actions can result in impacting professional standards as well as policy. The FCN must ensure that education and interventions provided be evidence based and applicable to the client. Aside from this, the FCN also has a responsibility to share research with other FCNs in meetings, conferences, and in publications. This exemplar illustrates how an FCN may fulfill this ethical role from scholarly inquiry to conducting research and, ultimately, sharing the findings of these activities with other FCNs, as well as nurses in other settings.

The FCN desired to assist members of the community in coping with the feelings of being overwhelmed by a new diagnosis. Through the FCN's own experience with terminally ill parents, specific elements seemed to ease these feelings and make provider appointments more organized, improve family communication, and reduce patients' fatigue. The FCN relied on reputable sources such as CINAHL and MEDLINE to explain helpful interventions. This review of literature indicated that improved communication, increased assertiveness, and decision-making helped patients deal more effectively with the consequences of a terminal illness.

The FCN developed a pilot project named New Diagnosis Toolkit. Persons from the community newly diagnosed, or with a family member with a new diagnosis, were provided a bag with specific tools and instructions for use. The contents of the kit included some prayer cards, a calendar, a tape recorder, a notebook, a folder, a blank medication list, and a pen. Participants were encouraged to write down questions, document all current meds and details of their regimens, and make a list of all healthcare providers seen and diagnostic tests completed, as well as indicate key dates on the calendar. Medical appointments were recorded so the patient and family could listen again after the encounter. Family members unable to attend appointments also listened to the cassettes instead of the ill family member needing to recall the details of the visit for later conversations. A month later, the participants and families were interviewed with questions specifically focused on anxiety, frustration, hope, and quality of family interactions. Patients reported feeling more organized, less stressed, and reported improved family relationships and less fatigue following appointments.

This FCN's development of a project to assist members of a faith community cope with new medical diagnoses has the potential to be incorporated in a variety of settings beyond the faith community. It can be formulated into a formal research project, published in a peer-reviewed journal to reach a larger audience, resulting in subsequent opportunities for replication. It has the potential to become a standard of faith community nursing practice.

Provision 8
The nurse collaborates with other health professionals and the public to protect and promote human rights, health diplomacy, and health initiatives.

An FCN employed by a regional healthcare system serves as a program manager, working with multiple faith community groups to promote health of body, mind, and spirit. In developing relationships with leaders in faith communities, the healthcare system, and the greater community, it became evident that significant health disparities exist within the community. The overall poverty rate is 26%, but some census tracts are rated 100% in poverty. These individuals have limited access to health care and frequently use the local emergency room as their only source of care. Data highlight significant disparities throughout the life span. The FCN participated in multiple discussions with various stakeholders. Simultaneously, the FCN assisted faith communities in developing health ministry programs, focusing on whole-person health with an emphasis on health promotion and disease prevention. Faith community members became empowered to make choices related to behaviors that impact health but consistently verbalized frustration at the lack of access to primary care and other resources.

As community and health system leaders continued to collaborate, the idea of a new community access network was developed. At the request of the designated leader, the FCN was invited to convene a group of residents who reside in the poorest census tracts and/or have their home faith community in those locales. Every person invited responded with enthusiasm. Monthly meetings are well attended. The designated leader of the new network presents updates and garners input from this advisory group regarding practice and policies as the network is built. Funds for a physical building were donated by a local foundation and the healthcare system, and construction is underway in one of the poorest census tracts. The advisory group participated in naming the new facility. As the structure is built, employees are being recruited from the neighborhoods that will be most impacted. The FCN continues to be a liaison between faith communities, the healthcare system, the new network, and the greater community. Because of established relationships, the FCN serves as an advocate and a voice, protecting and promoting human rights, striving for health equity for all.

Provision 9
The profession of nursing collectively through its professional organizations, must articulate nursing values, maintain the integrity of the profession, and integrate principles of social justice into nursing and health policy.

The role of a professional association is to help nurses maintain a healthy profession that advocates for the healthcare consumer, nurses, and society's trust. Professional associations are essential for generating the ideas, and proactive efforts needed to maintain professional practice. The values are articulated through the association's mission, vision, and standards of practice, educational activities, research, and other resources. The HMA is the voice for FCNs through its membership constituents, regional networks, national conference, annual meeting and ongoing collaboration with healthcare association allies. The HMA supports FCNs in regard to standards in nursing education, competency in nursing practice, personal spiritual development, and delivery of optimal whole-person patient care.

Faith community nurses are in advocacy roles for quality practices at the local, regional, and national levels. One way for FCNs to communicate consistent quality care and improve patient outcomes is by participating in collaborative projects through membership in their professional organizations. The result is a strong framework for effective communication and collaboration across denominations, community agencies, government entities, and healthcare disciplines.

The HMA is dedicated to reducing disease caused by tobacco use and exposure to secondhand smoke. One example of collaboration is the ongoing partnership that HMA has with the Centers for Disease Control and Prevention(CDC). This partnership includes the CDC's National Center for Chronic Disease Prevention and Health Promotion, the Office of Smoking and Health, and the CDC's Media Vendor, the Plowshare Group. The HMA brings comprehensive tobacco prevention information to its membership constituents through this collaborative partnership.

Through strategic efforts of this partnership, initiatives have been implemented to support tobacco control priorities by reaching out to faith communities and faith-related agencies nationwide.

The scope of work in HMA's partnership with the Office of Smoking and Health Partnership includes planning, implementation, and education for HMA's membership constituency and faith leaders nationwide. HMA is responsible for communicating timely, relevant information and education to constituents, faith leaders, faith communities, and partnering agencies. Specific initiatives include educational articles, smoking cessation stories shared by members for publication on the organization's website, participation in CDC's Smokefree Day Facebook event, and promotion of the Surgeon General's report on E-Cigarettes and Youth.

For over a decade, HMA has partnered with the Tobacco Free Kids Campaign. More recently, this movement transitioned to Faith United Against Tobacco. The HMA has followed goals for the initiative and emphasized the important role of FCNs working with faith leaders to advocate for policy change to reverse the tobacco epidemic. Participants have engaged in analyzing policy options that positively impacted houses of faith, such as implementing policies and procedures for Tobacco-Free Campuses while using a whole-person health approach.

Culturally Congruent Care

Culture refers to the learned, shared, and transmitted values, beliefs, norms, and life practices of a particular group that guide thinking, decisions, and actions in patterned ways (Leininger, 1995). Culture must be understood through cultural knowledge, cultural awareness, cultural encounters, and cultural skill (Campinha-Bacote, 2011). Nurses integrate cultural knowledge into practice when assessing, communicating with, and providing care for members of a racial, ethnic, or social group. This cultural expertise requires that the nurse has self-awareness of personal cultural identity, heritage, and values as well as engagement in lifelong learning to understand the culture of others (ANA, 2015b, p. 32). Through these stages of relationship building and interaction, the nurse must recognize and eliminate barriers to care that have been created by cultural differences.

Cultures may incorporate folk medicine practices and faith healing in their approaches to health and healing. Descriptive terminology specific to the culture may describe causes of illness and approaches for healing. One example is the Hispanic theory of disease, where ailments are thought to develop as a result of an imbalance between two humors: hot and cold. Consequently, the medications, remedies, and foods that are used to treat them are assigned descriptors accordingly. Leininger (2002) refers to these as *generic care systems*, which are folk practices defined culturally. Children who no longer live within their dominant culture may be conflicted in their approaches to health and well-being as they struggle to find a balance between the two cultures. The FCN serves to facilitate communication between generic system beliefs and treatment modalities and those of healthcare systems.

Faith community nurses advocate for appropriate levels of care for culturally diverse and vulnerable populations with limited access to healthcare resources. This may include refugee communities and other culturally linked communities. The FCN advocates for culturally congruent care that improves access to health care, promotes positive outcomes, and reduces disparities. Faith community nurses, aware of the impact of discrimination within and among vulnerable cultural groups, advocate for culturally sensitive care, which may include the use of medical interpreters and translators. Faith community nurses foster environments of civility, kindness, and respect for these members of society.

Educational Preparation for Faith Community Nursing
Faith Community Nurse

The FCN bridges two domains and therefore must be prepared in and responsible for both professional nursing practice and spiritual care. Some faith traditions may require additional educational stipulations and requirements.

The preferred minimum preparation for an RN or APRN entering the specialty of faith community nursing includes the following:

- Baccalaureate or higher degree in nursing with academic preparation in community-focused or population-focused care,
- Current experience as an RN using the nursing process,
- Knowledge of the healthcare assets and resources of the community,
- Specialized knowledge of the spiritual beliefs and practices of the faith community, and
- Specialized knowledge and skills to enable implementation of *Faith Community Nursing: Scope and Standards of Practice, Third Edition.*

With many FCNs practicing in autonomous settings, it is essential for this nursing specialty to support the 2010 Institute of Medicine's Future of Nursing Report recommendation that the proportion of nurses with baccalaureate degrees be increased to 80% by 2020 (IOM, 2010).

Appropriate and effective practice as an FCN requires the ability to integrate current nursing, behavioral, environmental, and spiritual knowledge with the unique spiritual beliefs and religious practices of the faith community into a program of whole-person care. Such integrative practice is required within all levels of the academic education of the nurse. With education, mentoring, and a collaborative practice site, an FCN may progress in expertise from novice to expert in this specialty practice.

Graduate-Level-Prepared RN

Graduate-level-prepared RNs are RNs prepared at the master's or doctoral educational level; have advanced knowledge, skills, abilities, and judgment; function in an advanced level as designated by elements of the nurse's position; and are not required to have additional regulatory oversight (ANA, 2015b, p. 2). Faith community nurses with graduate-level preparation may serve as faculty, adjunct faculty, or clinical preceptor at schools of nursing with responsibility for course development, research, and clinical oversight in courses associated with community health, spirituality content, and palliative care. Others may be administrators of healthcare systems' community outreach programs partnered with faith communities. Graduate-level-prepared RNs may also have leadership roles on boards of faith-based community agencies, provide consultative services, and serve as pastoral counselors or coordinators of missionary programs.

Advanced Practice Registered Nurse

By definition, an *advanced practice registered nurse* is a nurse

- Who has completed an accredited graduate-level education program preparing her or him for the role of certified nurse practitioner (CNP), certified registered nurse anesthetist (CRNA), certified nurse-midwife (CNM), or clinical nurse specialist (CNS);

- Who has passed a national certification examination that measures APRN-, role-, and population-focused competencies and maintain continued competence as evidenced by recertification in the role and population through the national certification program;

- Who has acquired advanced clinical knowledge and skills preparing the nurse to provide direct care to patients, as well as a component of indirect care; however, the defining factor for all APRNs is that a significant component of the education and practice focuses on direct care of individuals;

- Whose practices build on the competencies of RNs by demonstrating a greater depth and breadth of knowledge, a greater synthesis of data, increased complexity of skills and interventions, and greater role autonomy;

- Who is educationally prepared to assume responsibility and accountability for health promotion and/or maintenance as well as the assessment, diagnosis, and management of patient problems, which includes the use and prescription of pharmacologic and nonpharmacologic interventions;

- Who has clinical experience of sufficient depth and breadth to reflect the intended license;

- Who has obtained a license to practice as an APRN in one of the four APRN roles: certified registered nurse anesthetist (CRNA), certified nurse midwife (CNM), clinical nurse specialist (CNS), or certified nurse practitioner (CNP) (ANA, 2015b, pp. 2–3; APRN Joint Dialogue Group, 2008).

An emerging role in healthcare delivery models is that of an APRN and other graduate-level-prepared nurses who have also acquired additional specialized education for practice as an FCN. These nurses integrate theoretical and evidence-based knowledge from graduate nursing education with the specialized education of an FCN regarding the structure, spiritual beliefs, and practices of the faith group. Examples that illustrate this role include a nurse practitioner in a faith-based healthcare site, an oncology CNS, a palliative care CNS, and a mental health CNS practicing in a faith-based community clinic. Besides providing nursing care, these APRNs influence nursing care outcomes by serving as an advocate, consultant, or researcher in the specialty area; by providing expert consultation for spiritual leaders and other healthcare providers; and by identifying and facilitating improvements in health and wellness care.

Additional Faith-Related Designations

National leaders of faith groups that recognize the importance of integrating this specialty nursing practice into faith communities have developed mechanisms for mentoring and providing informal and formal education in concepts of spiritual beliefs, practices, and rituals. When such mechanisms are available within the faith group, the FCN may work with the leadership of the faith community to meet the additional educational and practice requirements to earn formal designation as a spiritual leader in the particular faith group.

Faith groups have different ways of designating or titling individuals who have attained an advanced level of preparation and often undergone examination to determine fitness for providing spiritual care. Faith care nurses who achieve the requirements defined by the faith group in which they are practicing may then be given a title by the faith community indicating their achievement, such as *deacon, minister of health,* or *pastoral associate.* Titles such as these have a specialized meaning within the faith community served and acknowledge the additional education and training received by the FCN specific to the faith tradition.

Educational Approaches

Currently, the education of all nursing students preparing for the national examination for RN licensure includes basic content on spiritual care. However, because of the intentional focus on spiritual care by the FCN, this educational exposure is not adequate preparation for assuming the specialty role of an FCN. Faith community nursing requires an extensive global knowledge base, which has led to the development of its own body of knowledge beyond that established for general professional nursing practice. Current and historically relevant documents are archived by HMA and the Westberg Institute. This body of knowledge is continuously evolving; education beyond that required for licensure is therefore necessary to ensure safe, quality faith community nursing practice. Faith community nursing is unique in that there are various educational entries into the specialty practice. Preparation may occur through accredited CE programs, baccalaureate courses, graduate nursing courses, or related content in counseling, public health, and pastoral care.

A CE foundational curriculum was developed in 1996 as a pilot project of Advocate Health Care and the Parish Nurse Resource Center (IPNRC) with collaboration among representatives from the existing leaders and educators of the emerging parish nursing community. A CE curriculum was developed for both the entry-level FCN and FCN program coordinator. That curriculum continues to be revised and offered under the leadership of the Westberg Institute for Faith Community Nursing (formerly IPNRC) and Church Health Center and through their relationship with numerous educational partners as classroom and online models (Church Health Center, 2017, https://church-health.org/).

In addition to the IPNRC curriculum, university-based CE and graduate degree curricula and certificate programs were developed at universities across the nation. Some examples include Marquette University, Georgetown University, Duke University, Concordia College, and Concordia University-Wisconsin. Faith denominations have also developed educational content specific to their faith practices and beliefs. These foundational courses provide solid entry-level educational preparation into the specialty. The HMA supports curricula development through active participation of content experts (http://hmassoc.org/).

Some FCNs have also completed graduate-level and doctoral-level preparation in clinical nursing specialties, complementary care, palliative care, and holistic care. Others have completed graduate-level course work in seminaries and schools of theology and religion and formal Clinical Pastoral Education. These interdisciplinary approaches to education and skill development expand FCNs' expertise and enhance their incorporation of spiritual care into their faith community nursing practice.

Mentoring

The American Association of Colleges of Nursing (AACN) position statement, *The Baccalaureate Degree in Nursing as Minimal Preparation for Professional Practice*, notes that health care is shifting from hospital-centered inpatient care to more primary and preventive care in communities. This requires nurses to function with more independence in clinical decision-making, case management, guiding patients through the maze of healthcare resources, and educating patients on treatment regimens and adoption of healthy lifestyles (AACN, 2000, p. 1).

Nurses moving from acute, inpatient settings into community-based faith community nursing practice require reflective self-assessment to identify individual learning needs and goals for gaining this greater degree of independence in a broader clinical setting. Mentoring during orientation can enhance faith community nursing practice.

Many FCNs begin their role as a lone practitioner without benefit of a health system or network to provide a nurturing environment for growth and development both spiritually and professionally. The novice FCN needs guidance and support in order to establish and sustain a successful professional practice. Mentoring programs can assist FCNs in competence development after completing foundational education. Linking the novice FCN with an experienced FCN can facilitate the sharing of knowledge, experiences, and wisdom and encourage growth and achievement by providing an open and supportive learning environment.

Spiritual Educational Preparation

Faith communities understand and often financially support CE and spiritual development for FCNs to enhance their ability to provide spiritual care. Educational institutions that specialize in religious education may offer relevant courses or programs of study focusing on spiritual support and care. Graduate courses may include master's degrees in Pastoral Studies, Spiritual Direction, Pastoral Counseling, and Religious Studies with a Concentration in Spirituality and Wellness. Interprofessional collaboration provides other opportunities to increase knowledge and skills, particularly related to spiritual care and population health.

Experiential and informal learning related to spirituality also enhances FCN competency. Use of small group approaches to theological reflection, shared verbatim writing exercises, and discussion of practice exemplars facilitate application of spiritual concepts. Individualized spiritual development can be guided through an ongoing interaction with a spiritual director (Chase-Ziolek, M, 2017). The FCN may also access social networks, platforms, and blogs for discussions focused on spirituality.

Certification Process by Portfolio

Certification is a voluntary process for FCNs who meet the eligibility require-ments and provides an opportunity for FCNs to document their achievement within their specialty practice. The ANCC now offers Certification by Portfolio in Faith Community Nursing. The HMA has supported professional nursing practice in faith community nursing through its development of standards of practice and an ongoing goal of developing formal recognition of competency through certification. Faith community nurses are encouraged to achieve certi-fication (http://nursecredentialing.org/FaithCommunityNursing).

In July 2013, HMA posted a call for those interested in participating in the ANCC Certification process to apply to the ANCC invitation. A Content Expert Panel met in Silver Spring, Maryland, that autumn. These candidates were selected by ANCC from the pool of applicants who responded to the ANCC invitation to serve in the certification process. In December 2013, an External Validation Committee was selected from the pool of applicants to review faith community nursing material compiled by the Content Expert Panel. This committee completed an in-depth survey. A Standard Setting Panel and Appraisers were selected by ANCC. In August 2014, ANCC launched the Portfolio Process for Certification for the Specialty Practice of Faith Commu-nity Nursing.

The designated credential for ANCC certification in faith community nursing is RN-BC. FCN is an abbreviation for *faith community nurse* and is not meant to indicate a credential. The abbreviation FCN should not be written following a nurse's name in a signature line. When certified, the FCN places RN-BC behind his or her name and then spells out faith community nursing to indicate the specialty.

Maintenance of certification beyond the initial certification examination is required every 5 years. Recertification requirements include a combination of professional practice hours and activities, such as CE credits/contact hours, program development, project implementation, publication, research, teaching (e.g., clinical precepting and CE presentations), academic education, and par-ticipation in professional organizations.

Ongoing Education and Competence

The ANA identifies aspects of competence and describes types of learning related to the practice of nursing: "Competence can be defined, measured and evaluated. Competence is situational, dynamic, and is both an outcome and an ongoing process. Competency is an expected level of performance that integrates knowledge, skills, abilities, and judgment in formal, informal, and reflective learning experiences. Knowledge encompasses thinking, understanding of science and humanities, professional standards of practice, and insights gained from practical experiences, personal capabilities, and leadership performance" (ANA, 2014).

"Formal learning most often occurs in structured, academic, and professional development environments, while informal learning can be described as experiential insights gained in work, community, home, and other settings. Reflective learning represents the recurrent thoughtful personal self-assessment, analysis, and synthesis of strengths and opportunities for improvement" (ANA, 2014).

Key requirements for FCNs include ongoing education, developing competencies, and maintaining competencies. Faith community nurses practice in the role of independent and collaborative direct care provider, educator, administrator, healthcare consultant, resource person, supervisor of support personnel, public relations representative, leader, and advocate. Faith community nurses integrate cognitive, psychomotor, communication, interpersonal, and diagnostic skills. Their ability to act effectively involves active listening, integrity, knowledge of one's strengths and weaknesses, positive self-regard, emotional intelligence, spiritual formation, and openness to feedback.

Faith community nurses must continually reassess their competencies and identify needs for additional knowledge, skills, personal growth, and integrative learning experiences (ANA, 2014). Competence in faith community nursing practice must be evaluated by the individual nurse, peers, mentors, and faith community leaders. No single evaluation method or tool can guarantee competence. Regardless of specialty, role, or setting, the RN remains accountable for the nursing care provided in their practice and addressing their own learning needs. This is of particular importance for all FCNs who generally work independently in the community setting.

Continued Commitment to the Profession

Because the specialty practice of faith community nursing is relatively small in numbers, each FCN is called upon to educate nurses, other healthcare providers, faith community leaders, and the general public about this nursing specialty. The FCN commits to lifelong learning in nursing, spiritual growth, and the beliefs and practices of the faith community. There are numerous opportunities for personal and professional growth in and beyond the community. Faith denominations support both programs and professional development. The HMA and other nursing organizations, as well as other disciplines, provide opportunities for professional networking and ongoing education in the practice specialty. While the FCN may be the only healthcare provider in the faith community, the best practice cannot be provided in isolation. Personal and professional support, education opportunities, and resources are available. Accessing these will improve both the care provided to the faith community and the continued progress of the specialty.

Research and Faith Community Nursing

Research studies that describe the scope of practice and evaluate benefits of faith community nursing specialty practice are increasing. Quantitative investigations derive statistically significant findings related to measurement of clinical outcomes and cost–benefits of faith community nursing interventions (Brown, Coppola, Giacona, Petriches, & Stockwell, 2009; Schroepfer, 2016; Yeaworth & Sailors, 2014). Descriptive studies illustrate relevant aspects of spiritual assessment, faith formation, and intentional whole-person care through use of interviews, focus groups, narratives, and observation of faith community nursing models of practice. Nursing theoretical frameworks and models for nursing evolved in the mid and late 20th century. Spiritual care has been an integral aspect of many nursing theories (Newman, 1995; Roy, 1976; Watson, 1985). Faith community nurses incorporate nursing theories and evidence-based findings as rationale for their nursing practice and interventions.

Every FCN is responsible to document their interventions and outcomes so the impact of this specialty can be measured accurately and contribute to future research efforts. While there has been growth in publications related to faith community nursing, it is critical to continue research and development of collaborative studies through shared data collection. Faith community nurses are encouraged to find opportunities to develop or participate in small-scale studies and pilot studies that may later be replicated in larger studies. These expanded evidence-based research studies have the potential to more accurately define, strengthen, and change faith community nursing.

Faith community nurses incorporate research findings on the spiritual dimensions of diagnosis, interventions, and outcomes to improve whole-person health for individuals, families, and communities. Research reports may be found in the nursing literature and publications of other health professionals, as well as the professional literature focused on health ministry, chaplaincy, theology, spirituality, and spiritual care. Findings from a variety of nonnursing disciplines provide understanding of the strong connection between spiritual well-being, participation in religious practices, and health. Research conducted at the National Institutes of Health and academic institutions has established a relationship between spiritual practices and health, thereby expanding the knowledge base for the specialty of faith community nursing (Asomugha, Derose, & Lurie 2011; Koenig, 2012). Involvement in a faith community provides health benefits through social support, a social identity, and a sense of power beyond one's self. Religious and spiritual practices, such as meditation, prayer, social connection, and touch, are reported to lengthen life, improve the quality of life, and improve health outcomes by enhancing psychological, physical, and spiritual well-being (Puchalski, 2012; Tay, Tan, Diener, and Gonzalez, 2013).

Faith community nurses in Doctorate of Philosophy (PhD) or Doctorate of Nursing Practice (DNP) degree programs and other graduate degree programs are conducting research and/or developing scholarly projects related to this specialty. The importance of research to this nursing specialty includes academic, clinical, and community settings. Faith community nurses participate in discovery of research questions and formulation of research studies related to the intersection of spirituality, theology, and health. Faith community nurses also share peer-reviewed findings with colleagues and integrate evidence-based research in their practice.

Research and theory articles about faith community nursing and related topics (spirituality and health, religion and health, religion, and spirituality) may be found in journals that address issues of cancer, aging, culture, behavioral health, alternative and complementary medicine, and community health in particular. Databases such as PUBMED, CINAHL, and MEDLINE may also be used for search of literature. Key search words may include *aging, behavioral health, caring, community health nursing, evidence-based practice, faith community nursing, holistic care, person-centered care, parish nursing, spirituality,* and *wholistic care.*

Faith community nurses have the potential to make significant contributions to research, which defines both the art and science of nursing. Documentation that describes interventions and resulting outcomes contributes to defining the impact and significance of faith community nursing. This nursing specialty abounds with future research opportunities.

Professional Trends and Issues in Faith Community Nursing

In the coming years, all nurses will experience the impact of emerging trends and challenges related to nursing practice and healthcare delivery. Faith community nurses have a professional responsibility to participate in examining potential and real impacts of change, developing positive productive responses, and evaluating outcomes. The ANA 2013 Membership Assembly conducted an electronic environmental scan completed by the nurses in attendance that envisioned future change impacting nursing and healthcare. The most frequently cited areas of future change included societal/external trends that will impact nursing, ways in which nurses are working differently, and ways in which patients are acting in new or different ways related to health (ANA, 2013).

The Value of Faith Community Nursing in Population Health

Faith community nurses bring great value to population health management. The FCN focuses on assessment and management of the physical, biological, spiritual, social, psychological, and environmental influences on health. Within the healthcare system, FCNs increasingly serve as the critical contact with and advocate for patients, families, and communities. "As the largest of the health professions, nursing plays a key role in enhancing the responsiveness of the healthcare system to the needs of all individuals and populations" (AACN, 2016). Faith community nurses are in an excellent position to identify issues affecting the health and well-being of their patients, discern patterns across patient populations, link patients with community resources and social services, and develop broad-based interventions (Bachrach & Thomas, 2016).

Faith community nurses integrate community involvement and knowledge about an entire population with personal, clinical understandings of the health and illness experiences of individuals and families within the population. Faith community nurses translate knowledge from the health and social sciences to individuals and population groups through targeted interventions, programs, and advocacy. They translate and articulate the health and illness experiences of diverse, often vulnerable, individuals and families in the population and assist members of the community to voice their problems and aspirations. Faith community nurses are knowledgeable about multiple strategies for intervention, from those applicable to the entire population to those for the faith community, the family, and the individual.

Faith Community Nursing Compared to Public Health and Home Health Nursing

The roles of faith community, home health, and public health nurses overlap in several functions and there are important distinctions. These specialties promote health and wellness through assessment of health status, planning, intervention, and evaluation of the outcome of care. Public health nurses, home health nurses, and FCNs provide education, referral to other healthcare providers, coordination of care, and advocacy for the healthcare consumer.

Public health and home health nursing are regulated by federal and state requirements for physician-ordered skilled home health care provided by an RN that is goal directed in treatment of disease. The healthcare consumer receives care at home on an intermittent basis until the goal is met. Reimbursement for care is provided through Medicare and third-party payers during the time frame in which skilled care is needed (Skemp, Dreher, & Lehmann, 2016). Most often, the patient is required to be homebound to qualify for service. Examples of skilled care include assessment of the patient's condition, teaching the patient and/or family how to administer medication or understand the disease process, administering treatments, and reporting changes in condition to the physician.

The FCN is able to provide care beyond the episode of insurance-based or Medicare skilled reimbursable need particularly performing the independent functions of nursing licensure. Faith community nurses presently are not reimbursed under Medicare or third-party payers. Faith community nurses provide ongoing spiritual care, supportive services, presence, and linkage with faith community resources such transportation to medical appointments regardless of homebound status or reimbursable skilled need (Hickman, 2006, p. 30). These supportive services are valuable in reducing hospital readmission rates and helping healthcare consumers manage their chronic conditions. The FCN is an accessible, constant, trusted source for health information and support that, in collaboration with other healthcare providers, serves the healthcare consumer to enhance whole-person health. The FCN bridges care between the faith-based system and the acute healthcare system providing health promotion, urgent care facilitation, referrals for services, and support for aging in place (Schroepfer, 2016).

Faith community nursing also differs from public health and home health nursing in the broader setting of practice of the FCN, which includes an individual, family, faith community, community-at-large, and population focus. Public health nursing typically focuses on the community as a whole including the social and physical environment and the social organizations in place to work toward improving health and protecting the health of the population. Public health interventions are often at a systems level in contrast to the more frequent individual or faith community interventions of the FCN (Skemp et al., 2016).

Faith community nurses frequently collaborate with public health and home health nurses to implement public health promotion initiatives within communities of faith. For example, a workgroup of public health personnel and parish nurses in Wisconsin developed an Infection Control and Emergency Preparedness Toolkit for the faith community and prepared communities of faith to prevent the spread of disease (Reilly et al., 2011). Faith community nurses bring their knowledge of the traditions and values of religious traditions to the development and implementation of health promotion activities in faith-based settings. They use the public health department expertise and other community resources to implement health education programs. The community benefits from these collaborative approaches to improving health.

Faith community nursing activities, like those of public health nurses, include the following:

1. Assessing social determinants of health within a specific population

2. Evaluating health trends and risk factors of population groups and helping to determine priorities for targeted interventions

3. Working with communities or specific population groups within the community to develop targeted health promotion and disease prevention activities

4. Participating in assessing and evaluating health services to ensure that people are informed about available programs and services and assisted in the use of those services

5. Providing essential input to interdisciplinary programs that monitor, anticipate, and respond to public health problems in population groups (ANA, 2000).

Faith community nurses provide a critical link between health care and communities of faith and understanding health and illness as it is experienced in peoples' lives. This understanding is translated into action for the community, congregation, families, and individuals served. The FCN illustrates this role through surveillance and monitoring of disease trends within the community. Faith community nurses contribute to systems for monitoring crucial health status indicators such as environmentally caused illnesses, immunization levels, infant mortality rates, and communicable disease occurrence, in order to identify problems that threaten the public's health and develop effective interventions.

Accompanying Presence and Care in Life Transitions

The role of the FCN in providing care during life transitions embodies the practice and ministry of integrated whole-person care. These nursing interventions begin with the promotion of well-being and the goal of preventing disease and chronic conditions in order to sustain a balance and quality of the life experience. The FCN provides guidance through the recognition of health status, awareness of brokenness, and the potential for return to the optimum level of contribution to overall quality of community health. Faith community nurses focus on meeting the needs of anyone experiencing health challenges. Examples include the following:

- The woman preparing for the birth of her child,

- The person newly diagnosed with a chronic or untreatable condition,

- Chronically ill older adults,

- The adolescent struggling for personal identity, and

- The person seeking employment in order to keep his/her family together.

All of these persons are in transition and each from time to time may seek acceptance, an accompanying presence, supportive and restorative care, and resources from the FCN.

Many FCNs serve an important function of providing transitional care following hospitalization of members of their faith communities. Their activities include home visits and phone calls that assess the person's ability to manage his or her care, purchase and take medications correctly, and follow through on discharge instructions. Faith community nurses also provide transitional care to persons at increased risk of complications and readmission, which may include those with chronic illnesses, isolated elderly persons, persons with limited healthcare literacy, and individuals or families who have limited economic resources.

Recently, posthospital transitional care has become formalized. It includes a range of *time-limited* services and environments that *complement primary care* and are designed to ensure healthcare continuity and avoid preventable poor outcomes among *at risk* populations as they move from one level of care to another, among multiple providers and across settings (Naylor et al., 2011). This model for APRNs includes interventions that may decrease or prevent readmission by providing comprehensive nursing interventions. This listing is similar to interventions that FCNs have provided:

- Review of the written discharge plan;

- Assessment of patient and/or caregiver understanding;

- Medication reconciliation;

- Postdischarge services: follow-up appointments, outstanding tests;

- Patient education: care procedures, safety, signals for contacting provider, what to do if problems arise;

- Telephone reinforcement; and

- Access to community resources and services.

Examples of healthcare-system-based models partnering with FCNs for transitional care are emerging. New payment policies have been enacted to encourage improved transitions by healthcare systems (Agency for Healthcare

Research and Quality, 2014). Shared reimbursement to FCNs is an area for ongoing inquiry and delineation when healthcare systems collaborate with FCNs to provide transitional care.

New models for healthcare delivery and reimbursement are being developed. In the next 2 to 5 years, reimbursement will shift from volume-driven fee-for-service to value-based models using metrics such as quality and patient satisfaction. Medicare's value-based modifier for large medical practices treating Medicare patients went into effect in 2015, with full implementation scheduled for 2017. One component of growing importance to patient satisfaction scores includes meeting emotional needs through spiritual assessment and care (Balboni et al., 2014; Williams, Meltzer, Arora, Chung, & Curlin, 2011). Patients whose spiritual needs are not being met are reporting lower ratings of quality and satisfaction with their care (Sharma, Astrow, Texeira, & Sulmasy, 2012). Nurses who address and support patient's spiritual needs can have a significant impact on patient satisfaction scores. This provides opportunity for FCNs, as experts in providing spiritual care, to collaborate with nursing education colleagues in providing spiritual care education to nurses in other specialties.

Behavioral Health/Mental Health Care

One in five adults in the United States is affected by mental illness in any given year. Mental illnesses occur across all ages, races, and income levels [National Alliance on Mental Illness (NAMI), 2016]. The American Psychiatric Association (APA, 2016) recognizes that religion and spirituality play a significant role in healing. Often those experiencing mental illnesses seek assistance from their faith leaders. Faith community nurses promote health of mind, body, and spirit and are in a unique position to support the mental health of individuals. The FCN provides interventions during times of stress and life transitions such as social support, health education, advocacy, and spiritual care to promote behavioral health (Anaebere & Delilly, 2012). The NAMI and the APA, along with faith leaders including FCNs, are advocating for welcoming and inclusive faith communities free of the stigma of mental illness. Many faith traditions are developing resources to assist faith communities in providing compassionate care for those with mental health concerns. Faith community nurses will assume leadership roles for the development of community-based mental health educational programs, advocate for increased funding and access to treatment centers, and promote supportive care for individuals and families living with mental illnesses.

Technology

Technology presents many benefits and challenges to every area of professional nursing practice, and must be used with forethought and intention. As we move into an increasingly technology-driven world, it is essential that faith community nursing is able to incorporate technical aspects into practice as well.

Electronic health records facilitate data capture and sharing, tracking quality measures, and patient access/control of their personal health data. Two position statements of ANA, "Electronic Health Record" and "Standardization and Interoperability of Health Information Technology: Supporting Nursing and the National Quality Strategy for Better Patient Outcomes," call for standardization and interoperability of health information technology (ANA, 2017). Efforts to simplify and standardize documentation have produced templates in automated charting systems. These formats have removed and/or restricted the use of free text, which excludes the patient's personal narrative from the standardized content of the EHR. Faith community nurses are encouraged to participate in modifications in EHR design, which will include increased free text space and enhance qualitative research and affirm the significant contribution of personal narrative.

Faith community nurses who practice in formal partnerships with healthcare systems contribute to EHR documentation. However, a significant number of FCNs practice independently in their faith communities. This results in gaps of essential data collection related to faith community nursing practice, which limits analysis of collective data and outcomes. It is essential to collect and analyze patient demographics and assessment information, nursing diagnoses, interventions, and outcome measurements in order to reflect the impact of the nursing care provided. Professional nursing organizations and networks are invited to participate with the specialty of faith community nursing in developing methods for collection of bundled data that will enable research and analysis while maintaining patient confidentiality.

Today, patients with chronic diseases, as well as those with interest in wellness and disease prevention, are using multiple forms of medical self-monitoring devices. This has changed the partnership between the patient and healthcare provider, putting more self-management decisions in the patient's control. The FCN provides education on monitoring devices, their cost versus benefit, and safety issues related to self-management. In this paradigm, the FCN works in a consulting case manager role, empowering patients to understand health conditions and monitor device data in relation to their desired health outcomes. The FCN guides users of self-monitoring devices to actively participate with their healthcare provider for a comprehensive approach to their health promotion and decision-making related to modifying interventions. The goal is for accurate and safe use of self-monitoring devices.

Technological advances in social media allow FCNs to connect on formal and informal platforms which allow for the sharing of ideas, connecting to peers, and discussing trends and concerns and questions related to faith community nursing practice. Because of the porous nature of social media, FCNs must be vigilant regarding "postings, images, recordings, or commentary which breaches their obligation to maintain and protect patient's rights to privacy and confidentiality" (ANA, 2015a, p. 9).

Telehealth Use

Technology can now help patients see specialists without leaving their communities, permit local providers to take advantage of distant expertise, and improve timeliness of care. Telemedicine initiatives typically are being launched to make existing healthcare activities more accessible and spread specialty coverage. Although telemedicine is often used to increase utilization, it may also be used to engage a population that is not receiving care and to introduce interventions and interactions that will catch health risks at an early stage.

The rising importance of certain types of care essential to an overall continuum of care—from behavioral health and home care to postacute—is creating opportunity for video-over-distance to make an impact (Health Resources Services Administration, 2016). Through use of various forms of telehealth available, the FCN has the opportunity to connect individuals and families to resources not previously available. The FCN facilitates the use of telehealth and its ongoing education and follow-up and continues to provide educational, clinical, and spiritual support as needed.

Compensation

The original model for faith community nursing was a grant-funded institutional model with nurses employed through a hospital organization and congregations sharing a portion of the costs associated with the nurses' services. Other structures evolved to meet the unique needs of communities and included the paid consortium model, the paid institutional model, the paid congregational model, and the unpaid congregational model. Over the years, these models continue to be most commonly used (Hickman, 2011).

Today, increasing numbers of FCNs are paid employees in their faith community nursing roles. Other FCNs are unpaid professionals in their faith community nursing roles. Whether paid or unpaid, an FCN is obligated to comply with the rules and regulations of professional nursing licensure and the standards of faith community nursing. It is common in faith communities to use the term *volunteer* for many nonprofessional roles such as lay health promoters and other care team members. The term *volunteer* is not preferred as a term to describe FCNs in an attempt to recognize the professional role of the nurse, even if unpaid. Therefore, the term *unpaid professional* is the preferred description for the role. Faith communities are engaged in establishing methods for financially supporting the work of FCNs. The compensation of an FCN may take on a variety of payment methods: from a salary in the most traditional sense to other forms of compensation, including CE conference fees, professional liability coverage, professional licensure and association fees, publication subscriptions, and other supportive resources.

Workplace Safety

The FCN routinely engages in health and wholeness assessment of individuals, families, faith communities, and the broader community for the purpose of prioritizing health-related needs. The FCN is an advocate for the protection of health and safety within culturally diverse and underserved, vulnerable populations. Identification of risk factors in the environment of the faith community location and structure are still within the scope of FCN practice (HMA/ANA, 2012). The geographical and geopolitical communities influence the health and safety of the FCN and the healthcare consumer. The FCN uses evidence-based practices to develop policy and procedures that address issues of safe access to facilities and personal and public safety in the event of an emergency. Emergency actions may include but are not limited to initiating first aid; using an automated external defibrillator (AED) or cardiopulmonary resuscitation (CPR); activating the local EMS; and contacting local authorities, family, friends, faith community resources, and social service agencies as mandated by law.

Workplace safety also applies to the environment in which the faith community practice occurs. This may include but is not limited to an individual's home, the faith community, and the community at large. Research has identified factors that may increase the risk of violence for some workers in certain worksites. Such factors include working alone or in isolated areas, providing services and care for those with behavioral health issues, and working in areas with high crime rates (Canadian Center for Occupational Health and Safety, 2016). By assessing their worksites, FCNs can reduce the likelihood of a safety-related incident. Well-written and implemented workplace safety policies and procedures combined with training can reduce the incidence of workplace violence in both the private sector and community. Maintenance of a safe work environment includes personal safety education for the FCN, with the awareness that both individual and healthcare consumers' safety is paramount.

Health Promotion and Self-Care

A growing trend is for people to assume active roles in preventive health. These may include self-care activities related to nutrition, exercise, and modifying environmental health risks. Self-care is not limited to those who are well. Persons with health problems are also taking a greater degree of responsibility in their care. Individuals are more knowledgeable about their health and their healthcare options. Health consumers are requesting more second opinions, demanding clear explanations, and reserving final decisions about diagnosis and treatment for themselves.

An Internet survey asked Internet users to whom did they turn for help, either online or offline, the last time they had a serious health issue (Pew Research Center, 2012). Responses indicated the following:

- 70% of U.S. adults got information, care, or support from a doctor or another healthcare professional;

- 60% of adults got information or support from friends and family; and

- 24% of adults got information or support from others who have the same health condition (Pew Research Center, 2012).

Accuracy of health information is essential. The FCN can assist the healthcare consumer to identify reliable printed and Internet sources of health and medical information, develop questions for healthcare provider appointments, and maintain a personal health history record. The FCN may oversee/facilitate faith-community-based support groups and health promotion by laity health promotors to assure appropriate educational processes suitable for various learning styles.

The professional nurse coach is an RN who integrates coaching competencies into any setting or specialty area of practice to facilitate a process of change or development that assists individuals or groups to realize their potential (ANA/AHNA, 2013). Faith community nurses are nurse coaches who guide health promotion initiatives for individuals, families, groups, and communities. Faith community nurses are participating in the Healthy People 2020 Initiative and the National Preventive Strategy. These programs empower individuals to make healthy choices and eliminate health disparities and also enable FCNs to contribute to data collection, research, and evaluation. In these coaching roles, FCNs will model the same health maintenance and health promotion measures they teach to promote their own well-being and health.

Summary of the Scope of Nursing Practice

Excellence in faith community nursing is promoted through active collaboration between HMA, the Westberg Institute for Faith Community Nursing, national not-for-profit and governmental associations promoting community health, healthcare systems, regional health ministry networks, seminaries, denominational associations, faith community nursing networks, and other nursing organizations related to this nursing specialty. This shared work defines the scope and standards of practice and associated competencies, develops relevant position statements related to concerns in practice, and promotes recognition of individual expertise through ANCC certification by portfolio in faith community nursing.

Advancement of this nursing specialty will be shaped through the commitment of individual FCNs actively participating in professional associations, maintaining competency in evolving nursing practice, documenting the impact of interventions and outcomes, conducting self-reflection, and pursuing lifelong learning. Faith community nurses are well poised to respond to the evolving needs of individuals, families, and communities in their pursuit of health and wellness.

An invitation is extended to nursing organizations, health ministry organizations, community health organizations, and faith denomination organizations to actively participate in advancing faith community nursing practice, research, and education. Collaborative conversations, shared educational programming, and inclusive visioning will unify the broad diversity within this specialty.

Standards of Faith Community Nursing Practice

The term *faith community nurse* is used to represent a licensed RN specializing in faith community nursing.

Standards of Practice for Faith Community Nursing

Standard 1. Assessment
The faith community nurse collects pertinent data and information relative to the healthcare consumer's health or the situation.

Competencies

The faith community nurse:

> ▶ Collects pertinent data, including but not limited to demographics, social determinants of health, health disparities, and physical, functional, psychosocial, emotional, cognitive, sexual, cultural, age-related, environmental, spiritual/transpersonal, and economic assessments in a systematic, ongoing process with compassion and respect for the inherent dignity, worth, and unique attributes of every person.

> ▶ Recognizes the importance of the assessment parameters identified by World Health Organization (WHO), Healthy People 2020, or other organizations that influence nursing practice.

> ▶ Integrates knowledge from global and environmental factors into the assessment process.

> ▶ Elicits the healthcare consumer's values, preferences, expressed and unexpressed needs, and knowledge of the healthcare situation.

- ▶ Recognizes the impact of one's own personal attitudes, values, and beliefs on the assessment process.
- ▶ Identifies barriers to effective communication based on psychosocial, literacy, financial, spiritual, religious, and cultural considerations.
- ▶ Assesses the impact of family dynamics on healthcare consumer health and wellness.
- ▶ Engages the healthcare consumer and other interprofessional team members, in culturally sensitive data collection related to health and wholeness.
- ▶ Prioritizes data collection based on the healthcare consumer's immediate condition or the anticipated needs of the healthcare consumer or situation.
- ▶ Uses evidence-based assessment techniques, instruments, tools, available data, information, and knowledge relevant to the situation to identify patterns and variances.
- ▶ Applies ethical, legal, and privacy guidelines and policies to the collection, maintenance, use, and dissemination of data and information.
- ▶ Recognizes the healthcare consumer as the authority on their own health by honoring their care preferences.
- ▶ Documents relevant data accurately and in a confidential manner and accessible to the interprofessional team when applicable.

Additional competencies for the graduate-level-prepared faith community nurse

In addition to the faith community nurse competencies, the graduate-level-prepared faith community nurse and the advanced practice faith community nurse:

- ▶ Assesses the effect of interactions among individuals, family, community, and social systems on health and illness.
- ▶ Synthesizes the results and information leading to clinical understanding.

Additional competencies for the advanced practice faith community nurse

In addition to the competencies of the faith community nurse and the graduate-level-prepared faith community nurse, the advanced practice faith community nurse:

- Initiates diagnostic tests and procedures relevant to the healthcare consumer's current status.

- Uses advanced assessment, knowledge, and skills to maintain, enhance, or improve health conditions.

Standard 2. Diagnosis

The faith community nurse analyzes assessment data to determine actual or potential diagnoses, problems, and issues.

Competencies

The faith community nurse:

- ▶ Identifies actual, perceived, or potential risks to the healthcare consumer's health and safety or barriers to health and wholeness, which may include but are not limited to interpersonal, systematic, cultural, spiritual, or environmental circumstances.

- ▶ Uses assessment data, standardized classification systems when available, technology, and clinical decision support tools to articulate actual or potential diagnoses, problems, and issues.

- ▶ Verifies the diagnoses, problems, and issues with the individual, family, group, spiritual leader, community, population, and interprofessional colleagues when possible and appropriate.

- ▶ Prioritizes diagnoses, problems, and issues based on mutually established goals to meet the needs of the healthcare consumer across the health–illness continuum.

- ▶ Documents diagnoses, problems, and issues in a manner that facilitates the determination of the expected outcomes and plan.

- ▶ Identifies strengths that enhance health and spiritual well-being.

Additional competencies for the graduate-level-prepared faith community nurse

In addition to the competencies of the faith community nurse, the graduate-level-prepared faith community nurse:

- ▶ Uses information and communication technologies to analyze diagnostic practice patterns of nurses and other members of the interprofessional healthcare team.

- ▶ Employs aggregate-level data to articulate diagnoses, problems, and issues of healthcare consumers and organizational systems.

Additional competencies for the advanced practice faith community nurse

In addition to the competencies of the faith community nurse and the graduate-level-prepared faith community nurse, the advanced practice faith community nurse:

▶ Formulates a differential diagnosis based on the assessment, history, physical examination, and diagnostic test results.

Standard 3. Outcomes Identification

The faith community nurse identifies expected outcomes for a plan individualized to the healthcare consumer or the situation.

Competencies

The faith community nurse:

- ▶ Engages the healthcare consumer, interprofessional team, family, spiritual leaders, and others in partnership to identify expected outcomes.

- ▶ Formulates culturally sensitive expected outcomes derived from assessments and diagnoses.

- ▶ Uses clinical expertise and current evidence-based practice to identify health risks, benefits, costs, and/or expected trajectory of the condition.

- ▶ Collaborates in supporting decision-making shared between the healthcare consumer and healthcare providers to define expected outcomes, integrating the individual's culture, spiritual and faith beliefs and practices, values, ethical considerations, environment, and current evidence-based practice.

- ▶ Generates a time frame for the attainment of expected outcomes.

- ▶ Develops expected outcomes that facilitate coordination of care.

- ▶ Develops expected outcomes that facilitate attaining, maintaining, or regaining health, healing, and hope.

- ▶ Modifies expected outcomes based on the evaluation of the status of the healthcare consumer and situation.

- ▶ Documents expected outcomes as measurable goals.

- ▶ Evaluates the actual outcomes in relation to expected outcomes, safety, and quality standards.

Additional competencies for the graduate-level-prepared faith community nurse, including the APRN

In addition to the competencies of the faith community nurse, the graduate-level-prepared faith community nurse or advanced practice faith community nurse:

▶ Defines expected outcomes that incorporate cost, clinical effectiveness, and are aligned with the outcomes identified by members of the interprofessional team.

▶ Differentiates outcomes that require care process interventions from those that require system-level actions.

▶ Integrates scientific evidence and best practices to achieve expected outcomes.

▶ Advocates for outcomes that reflect the healthcare consumer's culture, values, and ethical concerns.

Standard 4. Planning

The faith community nurse develops a plan that prescribes strategies to attain expected, measurable outcomes.

Competencies

The faith community nurse:

- ▶ Develops a whole-person-centered, evidence-based plan in partnership with the healthcare consumer, family, and interprofessional team that considers the person's characteristics or situation, but not limited to values, spiritual beliefs and practices, health practices, preferences, choices, developmental level, coping style, culture, religious rites, environment, and available technology.

- ▶ Establishes the plan priorities with the healthcare consumer, family, interprofessional team, and others, as appropriate.

- ▶ Advocates for responsible and appropriate use of interventions to minimize unwarranted or unwanted treatment and/or suffering of the individual.

- ▶ Prioritizes elements of the plan based on the assessment of the healthcare consumer's level of risk and safety needs.

- ▶ Includes evidence-based strategies in the plan to address each of the identified diagnoses, issues, and strengths. These strategies may include but are not limited to:

  - ▶ Promotion and restoration of health,

  - ▶ Spiritual enhancement,

  - ▶ Prevention of illness, injury, and disease,

  - ▶ Facilitation of healing,

  - ▶ Alleviation of suffering, and

  - ▶ Provision of supportive care

- ▶ Incorporates an implementation pathway that describes steps and milestones.

- ▶ Identifies cost and economic implications of the plan for healthcare consumer, family, caregivers, or other affected parties and how faith community resources and local community resources may be of assistance.

- ► Develops a plan that reflects compliance with current statutes, rules and regulations, and standards.
- ► Includes the synthesis of healthcare consumers' values and spiritual beliefs regarding nursing and medical therapies in the plan.
- ► Modifies the plan according to the ongoing assessment of the healthcare consumer's response and other outcome indicators.
- ► Documents the plan using standardized language or recognized terminology.
- ► Includes strategies for whole-person health, with a focus on spirituality and growth across the life span.

Additional competencies for the graduate-level-prepared RN

In addition to the competencies of the registered nurse, the graduate-level-prepared registered nurse:

- ► Incorporates assessment strategies, diagnostic strategies, and therapeutic interventions that reflect current evidence-based knowledge and practice for population health, as well as the health of individuals and families.
- ► Designs strategies and tactics to meet the multifaceted whole-person health and complex needs of healthcare consumers or others.
- ► Leads the design and development of interprofessional processes to address the identified diagnoses, problems, or issues.
- ► Designs innovative nursing practices.
- ► Actively participates in the development and continuous improvement of systems that support the planning process.

Additional competencies for the advanced practice registered nurse

In addition to the competencies of the registered nurse and graduate-level-prepared registered nurse, the advanced practice registered nurse:

- ► Integrates assessment strategies, diagnostic strategies, and therapeutic interventions that reflect current evidence-based knowledge and practice.

Standard 5. Implementation

The faith community nurse implements the identified plan.

Competencies

The faith community nurse:

▶ Partners with the healthcare consumer, family, and significant others to implement the plan in a safe, effective, efficient, timely, patient-centered, and equitable manner (IOM, 2010).

▶ Integrates interprofessional team partners including spiritual leaders, caregivers, and volunteers from diverse backgrounds in implementation of the plan through collaboration and communication across the continuum of care.

▶ Demonstrates caring behaviors toward healthcare consumers, significant others, and groups of people receiving care to develop therapeutic relationships necessary for health and healing.

▶ Provides culturally congruent, whole-person care that focuses on the healthcare consumer and addresses and advocates for the needs of diverse and vulnerable populations across the lifespan with particular emphasis on spiritual needs.

▶ Uses evidence-based interventions and strategies to achieve the mutually identified goals and outcomes specific to the problem or needs.

▶ Integrates critical thinking and technology solutions to implement the nursing process to collect, measure, record, retrieve, trend, and analyze data and information to enhance nursing practice and healthcare consumer, family, or population group outcomes.

▶ Delegates according to the health, safety, and welfare of the healthcare consumer and considering the circumstance, person, task, direction or communication, supervision, evaluation, as well as the state nurse practice act regulations, institution, and regulatory entities while maintaining accountability for the care.

▶ Uses community and faith community resources and systems to implement the plan.

▶ Documents implementation and any modifications, including changes or omissions, of the identified plan.

Additional competencies for the graduate-level-prepared faith community nurse

In addition to the competencies of the faith community nurse, the graduate-level-prepared faith community nurse:

▶ Uses systems in the faith community, organizations, and community resources to lead effective change and implement the plan.

▶ Applies quality principles while articulating methods, tools, performance measures, and standards as they relate to implementation of the plan.

▶ Translates evidence into practice to initiate change in faith community nursing care practices if desired outcomes are not achieved.

▶ Leads interprofessional teams to communicate, collaborate, and consult effectively.

▶ Demonstrates leadership skills that emphasize ethical and critical decision-making, effective working relationships, and a systems perspective.

▶ Serves as a consultant to provide additional insight and potential solutions.

▶ Uses theory-driven approaches in the development and continuous improvement of systems that support implementation of the plan.

Additional competencies for the advanced practice faith community nurse

In addition to the competencies of the faith community nurse and graduate-level-prepared faith community nurse, the advanced practice faith community nurse:

▶ Uses prescriptive authority, procedures, referrals, treatments, and therapies in accordance with state and federal laws and regulations.

▶ Prescribes traditional and integrative evidence-based treatments, therapies, and procedures that are compatible with the healthcare consumer's cultural preferences and norms.

▶ Prescribes therapies, including those that strengthen the body–mind–spirit connection such as meditation, prayer, guided imagery, and various rituals of worship.

▶ Prescribes evidence-based pharmacological agents and treatments according to clinical indicators and results of diagnostic and laboratory tests.

▶ Provides clinical consultation for healthcare consumers and professionals related to complex clinical cases to improve care and outcomes.

Standard 5A. Coordination of Care

The faith community nurse coordinates care delivery.

Competencies

The faith community nurse:

▶ Organizes the components of the plan.

▶ Collaborates with the consumer to help manage health care based on mutually agreed-upon outcomes.

▶ Coordinates implementation of a whole-person-centered plan of care with particular emphasis on the spiritual needs of diverse populations.

▶ Manages a healthcare consumer's care in order to maximize independence and quality of life in accordance with mutually agreed upon outcomes.

▶ Engages healthcare consumers in self-care to achieve preferred goals for quality of life with attention to mind, body, and spirit.

▶ Assists the healthcare consumer to identify options for care.

▶ Communicates with the healthcare consumer, family, interprofessional team, and community-based resources to effect safe transitions in continuity of care.

▶ Advocates for the delivery of dignified and whole-person humane care by the interprofessional team.

▶ Documents the coordination of care.

Additional competencies for the graduate-level-prepared faith community nurse

In addition to the competencies of the faith community nurse, the graduate-level-prepared faith community nurse:

▶ Provides leadership in the coordination of interprofessional health care for integrated delivery of healthcare consumer services to achieve safe, effective, efficient, timely, patient-centered, and equitable care (IOM, 2010).

- ▶ Provides leadership in advocating for the delivery of dignified and humane care.

- ▶ Coordinates system and community resources that enhance delivery of care across continuums.

Additional competencies for the advanced practice faith community nurse

In addition to the competencies of the faith community nurse and graduate-level-prepared faith community nurse, the advanced practice faith community nurse:

- ▶ Manages identified consumer panels or populations.

- ▶ Serves as the healthcare consumer's primary care provider and coordinator of healthcare services in accordance with state and federal laws and regulations.

- ▶ Synthesizes data and information to diagnose, prescribe and provide necessary system and community support measures, including modifications of environments.

Standard 5B. Health Teaching and Health Promotion

The faith community nurse employs strategies to promote health and a safe environment.

Competencies

The faith community nurse:

▶ Provides opportunities for the healthcare consumer to identify needed healthcare promotion, disease prevention, and self-management topics.

▶ Uses health promotion and health teaching methods in collaboration with the healthcare consumer's values, beliefs, health practices, developmental level, learning needs, readiness and ability to learn, language preference, spirituality, culture, and socioeconomic status.

▶ Uses feedback and evaluations from the healthcare consumer to determine the effectiveness of the employed strategies.

▶ Uses information technologies to communicate health promotion and disease prevention information to the healthcare consumer.

▶ Provides healthcare consumers with information about intended effects and potential adverse effects of the plan of care and proposed therapies.

▶ Engages consumer alliance and advocacy groups in health teaching and health promotion activities for healthcare consumers.

▶ Provides anticipatory guidance to healthcare consumers to promote health and prevent or reduce the risk of negative health outcomes.

▶ Teaches activities that strengthen the body–mind–spirit connection, such as meditation, prayer, and guided imagery.

▶ Evaluates health information resources for use in health community nursing for accuracy, readability, and comprehensibility by healthcare consumers and compatibility with the healthcare consumers' spiritual beliefs and practices.

Additional competencies for the graduate-level-prepared faith community nurse, including the APRN

In addition to the competencies of the faith community nurse, the graduate-level-prepared faith community nurse or advanced practice faith community nurse:

▶ Synthesizes empirical evidence on risk behaviors, gender roles, learning theories, behavioral change theories, motivational theories, translational theories for evidence-based practice, epidemiology, and other related theories and frameworks when designing health education information and programs.

▶ Evaluates health information resources for applicability, accuracy, readability, and comprehensibility to help healthcare consumers access quality health information that is compatible with their spiritual beliefs and practices.

▶ Engages faith-based organizations, consumer alliances, and advocacy groups, as appropriate, in health teaching and health promotion activities that are restorative, supportive, and promotive in nature.

▶ Provides anticipatory guidance to individuals, families, and groups in the faith community to promote health and prevent or reduce the risk of health problems.

Standard 6. Evaluation

The faith community nurse evaluates progress toward attainment of goals and outcomes.

Competencies

The faith community nurse:

- Conducts a systematic, ongoing, and criterion-based evaluation of the goals and outcomes in relation to the structure, processes, and timeline prescribed in the plan.

- Collaborates with the healthcare consumer and others involved in the care or situation in the evaluation process.

- Determines, in partnership with the healthcare consumer and other stakeholders, the patient-centeredness, effectiveness, efficiency, safety, timeliness, and equitability (IOM, 2001) of the strategies in relation to the responses to the plan and attainment of outcomes. Other defined criteria (e.g., Quality and Safety Education for Nurses) may be used as well.

- Demonstrates sensitivity to the complex dynamics of faith community settings.

- Uses ongoing assessment data to revise the diagnoses, outcomes, plan, and implementation strategies.

- Shares evaluation data and conclusions with the healthcare consumer and other stakeholders in accordance with federal and state regulations.

- Documents the results of the evaluation including results related to faith and spiritual realms.

Additional competencies for the graduate-level-prepared faith community nurse, including the APRN

In addition to the competencies of the faith community nurse, the graduate-level-prepared faith community nurse or the advanced practice faith community nurse:

- Uses tools to identify the influence of the healthcare consumer's and family's view of health and healing on the attainment of outcomes.

▶ Synthesizes evaluation data from the healthcare consumer, community, population and/or institution to determine the effectiveness of the plan.

▶ Engages in a systematic evaluation process to revise the plan to enhance its effectiveness.

▶ Uses results of the evaluation to make or recommend process, policy, procedure, or protocol revisions when warranted.

▶ Uses the results of the evaluation analyses to increase awareness beyond the individual faith community of the health and wellness benefits and spiritual care provided.

Standards of Professional Performance

Standard 7. Ethics
The faith community nurse practices ethically.

Competencies
The faith community nurse:

▶ Integrates the *Code of Ethics for Nurses with Interpretive Statements* (ANA, 2015a) to guide nursing practice and articulate the moral foundation of nursing.

▶ Practices with compassion and respect for the inherent dignity, worth, tenets of faith and spiritual beliefs, and unique attributes of all people.

▶ Advocates for healthcare consumers' rights to informed decision-making and self-determination.

▶ Seeks guidance in situations where the rights of the individual conflict with public health guidelines.

▶ Endorses the understanding that the primary commitment is to the healthcare consumer regardless of setting or situation.

▶ Maintains therapeutic relationships and professional boundaries.

▶ Recognizes the centrality of the healthcare consumer and family as core members of the healthcare team.

▶ Acknowledges and respects tenets of the faith and spiritual belief system of a healthcare consumer.

▶ Delivers care in a manner that preserves and protects the healthcare consumer's autonomy, dignity, rights, and spiritual beliefs and practices.

- Advocates for the rights, health, and safety of the healthcare consumer and others.
- Safeguards the privacy and confidentiality of healthcare consumers, others, and their data and information within ethical, legal, religious, and regulatory parameters.
- Demonstrates professional accountability and responsibility for nursing practice.
- Maintains competence through continued personal and professional development.
- Demonstrates commitment to self-reflection and self-care.
- Contributes to the establishment and maintenance of an ethical environment that is conducive to safe, quality health care.
- Advances the profession through scholarly inquiry, professional standards development, and the generation of policy.
- Collaborates with other health professionals and the public to protect human rights, promote health diplomacy, enhance cultural sensitivity and congruence, and reduce health disparities.
- Articulates nursing values to maintain personal integrity and the integrity of the profession.
- Integrates principles of social justice into nursing and policy.

Additional competencies for the graduate-level-prepared faith community nurse, including the APRN

In addition to the competencies of the registered nurse, the graduate-level-prepared faith community nurse:

- Participates in interprofessional teams that address ethical risks, benefits, and outcomes of programs and decisions that affect health and healthcare delivery.
- Mentors interprofessional teams in processes of ethical decision-making.
- Advocates for equitable healthcare consumer care.

Standard 8. Culturally Congruent Practice

The faith community nurse practices in a manner that is congruent with cultural diversity and inclusion principles.

Competencies

The faith community nurse:

- ▶ Demonstrates respect, equity, and empathy in actions and interactions with all healthcare consumers.
- ▶ Participates in lifelong learning to understand cultural preferences, worldview, choices, and decision-making processes of diverse consumers.
- ▶ Creates an inventory of one's own values, beliefs, and cultural heritage.
- ▶ Applies knowledge of variations in health beliefs and practices, religious tenets, and communication patterns in all nursing practice activities.
- ▶ Identifies the stage of the consumer's acculturation and accompanying patterns of needs and engagement.
- ▶ Considers the effects and impact of discrimination and oppression on practice within and among vulnerable cultural groups.
- ▶ Uses skills and tools that are appropriately vetted for the culture, literacy, and language of the population served.
- ▶ Communicates with appropriate language and behaviors, including the use of medical interpreters and translators in accordance with consumer preferences.
- ▶ Identifies the cultural-specific meaning of interactions, terms, and content.
- ▶ Respects consumer decisions based on age, tradition, belief and family influence, and stage of acculturation.
- ▶ Advocates for policies that promote whole-person health and prevent harm among culturally diverse, underserved, or underrepresented consumers.

- ▶ Promotes equal access to services, tests, interventions, health promotion programs, enrollment in research, education, and other opportunities.
- ▶ Educates nurse colleagues and other professionals about cultural similarities and differences of healthcare consumers, families, groups, communities, and populations.

Additional competencies for the graduate-level-prepared faith community nurse

In addition to the competencies of the faith community nurse, the graduate-level-prepared faith community nurse:

- ▶ Evaluates tools, instruments, and services provided to culturally diverse populations.
- ▶ Advances organizational policies, programs, services, and practice that reflect respect, equity, and values for diversity and inclusion.
- ▶ Engages consumers, key stakeholders, and others in designing and establishing internal and external cross-cultural partnerships.
- ▶ Conducts research to improve health care and healthcare outcomes for culturally diverse consumers.
- ▶ Develops recruitment and retention strategies to achieve a multicultural workforce.

Additional competencies for the advanced practice faith community nurse

In addition to the competencies of the faith community nurse and graduate-level-prepared faith community nurse, the advanced practice faith community nurse:

- ▶ Promotes shared decision-making solutions in planning, prescribing, and evaluating processes when the healthcare consumer's cultural preferences and norms may create incompatibility with evidence-based practice.
- ▶ Leads interprofessional teams to identify the cultural and language needs of the consumer.

Standard 9. Communication

The faith community nurse communicates effectively in all areas of practice.

Competencies

The faith community nurse:

- ▶ Assesses one's own communication skills and effectiveness.

- ▶ Demonstrates cultural empathy when communicating.

- ▶ Assesses communication ability, health literacy, resources, and preferences of healthcare consumers to inform the interprofessional team and others.

- ▶ Uses language translation resources to ensure effective communication.

- ▶ Incorporates appropriate alternative strategies to communicate effectively with healthcare consumers who have visual, speech, language, or communication difficulties.

- ▶ Uses communication styles and methods that demonstrate caring, respect, deep listening, authenticity, and trust.

- ▶ Conveys accurate information.

- ▶ Maintains communication with interprofessional team and others to facilitate safe transitions and continuity in care delivery.

- ▶ Contributes nursing and spiritual perspectives in interactions with others and discussions with the interprofessional team.

- ▶ Exposes care processes and decisions when they do not appear to be in the best interest of the healthcare consumer.

- ▶ Discloses concerns related to potential or actual hazards and errors in care or the practice environment to the appropriate level.

- ▶ Demonstrates continuous improvement of communication skills.

Additional competencies for the graduate-level-prepared faith community nurse, including the APRN

In addition to the competencies of the faith community nurse, the graduate-level-prepared faith community nurse or advanced practice faith community nurse:

> ▶ Assumes a leadership role in shaping or fashioning environments that promote healthy communication.

Standard 10. Collaboration

The faith community nurse collaborates with the healthcare consumer and other key stakeholders in the conduct of nursing practice.

Competencies

The faith community nurse:

- ▶ Identifies the areas of expertise and contribution of other professionals and key stakeholders.

- ▶ Clearly articulates the nurse's role and responsibilities within the team.

- ▶ Uses the unique and complementary abilities of all members of the team to optimize attainment of desired outcomes.

- ▶ Partners with the healthcare consumer and key stakeholders to advocate for and effect change, leading to positive outcomes and quality care.

- ▶ Communicates with the healthcare consumer, family, groups, spiritual leaders, hospital and hospice chaplains, and other healthcare providers regarding healthcare consumer care and the faith community nurse's role in the provision of that care.

- ▶ Uses appropriate tools and techniques, including information systems and technologies, to facilitate discussion and team functions, in a manner that protects dignity, respect, privacy, and confidentiality.

- ▶ Promotes engagement through consensus building and conflict management.

- ▶ Uses effective group dynamics and strategies to enhance team performance.

- ▶ Exhibits dignity and respect when interacting with others and giving and receiving feedback.

- ▶ Partners with all stakeholders to create, implement, evaluate, and document a comprehensive plan.

Additional competencies for the graduate-level-prepared faith community nurse, including the APRN

In addition to the competencies of the faith community nurse, the graduate-level-prepared faith community nurse, or advanced practice faith community nurse:

▶ Participates in interprofessional activities, including but not limited to education, consultation, management, technological development, or research to enhance outcomes.

▶ Invites the contribution of the healthcare consumer, family, and team members in order to achieve optimal outcomes.

▶ Provides leadership for establishing, improving, and sustaining collaborative relationships to achieve safe, quality care for healthcare consumers.

▶ Advances interprofessional plan-of-care documentation and communications, rationales for plan-of-care changes, and collaborative discussions to improve healthcare consumer outcomes.

▶ Participates on interprofessional teams that contribute to role development and, directly or indirectly, advance nursing practice and health services.

Standard 11. Leadership

The faith community nurse leads within the professional practice setting and the profession.

Competencies

The faith community nurse:

- ▶ Serves as a nursing role model in the establishment of an environment that supports and maintains respect, trust, and dignity.

- ▶ Encourages innovation in practice and role performance to attain personal and professional plans, goals, and vision.

- ▶ Communicates to manage change and address conflict.

- ▶ Mentors colleagues for the advancement of nursing practice, the profession, and the specialty of faith community nursing to enhance safe, quality health care.

- ▶ Retains accountability for delegated nursing care.

- ▶ Contributes to the evolution of the profession through participation in professional organizations, professional development, certification, and continuing education.

- ▶ Demonstrates a commitment to lifelong learning, education, and spiritual growth for self and others.

- ▶ Influences policies that promote health and improve healthcare consumer outcomes.

- ▶ Collaborates to create a compelling and inspiring vision of excellence in nursing practice within the organization and the community.

- ▶ Serves in key leadership roles in the faith community by participating on committees, councils, and health ministry administrative teams.

- ▶ Endorses nursing autonomy and accountability and establishes an environment that motivates constructive change.

Additional competencies for the graduate-level-prepared faith community nurse, including the APRN

In addition to the competencies of the faith community nurse, the graduate-level-prepared faith community nurse or advanced practice faith community nurse:

- ▶ Influences decision-making bodies to improve the professional practice environment and healthcare consumer outcomes.

- ▶ Enhances the effectiveness of the interprofessional team.

- ▶ Promotes advanced practice nursing and role development by interpreting its role for healthcare consumers and policy makers.

- ▶ Models expert practice to interprofessional team members and healthcare consumers.

- ▶ Mentors colleagues in the acquisition of clinical knowledge, skills, abilities, and judgment.

Standard 12. Education

The faith community nurse seeks knowledge and competence that reflects current nursing practice and promotes futuristic thinking.

Competencies

The faith community nurse:

- ▶ Identifies learning needs based on nursing knowledge and the various roles the nurse may assume and the changing needs of the population.

- ▶ Participates in ongoing educational activities related to nursing and interprofessional knowledge bases and professional topics and spiritual care.

- ▶ Mentors nurses new to their roles for the purpose of ensuring successful enculturation, orientation, and emotional support.

- ▶ Demonstrates a commitment to lifelong learning through self-reflection and inquiry for learning and personal growth.

- ▶ Seeks experiences that reflect current practice to maintain and advance knowledge, skills, abilities, attitudes, and judgment in clinical practice or role performance for faith community nursing.

- ▶ Acquires knowledge and skills relative to the role, population, specialty of faith community nursing, setting, and global or local health situation.

- ▶ Participates in formal consultations or informal discussions to address issues in nursing practice as an application of education and knowledge.

- ▶ Identifies modifications or accommodations needed in the delivery of education based on healthcare consumer and family members' needs.

- ▶ Shares educational findings, experiences, and ideas with peers.

- ▶ Supports acculturation of nurses new to their roles by role modeling, encouraging, and sharing pertinent information relative to optimal care delivery.

- ▶ Facilitates a work environment supportive of ongoing education of healthcare professionals.

- ▶ Maintains a professional portfolio that provides evidence of individual competence and lifelong learning.

Standard 13. Evidence-Based Practice and Research

The faith community nurse integrates evidence and research findings into practice.

Competencies

The faith community nurse:

▶ Articulates the values of research and its application relative to the healthcare setting and practice.

▶ Identifies questions in the healthcare setting and practice as well as the spirituality, theology, and health intersection that can be answered by nursing research.

▶ Uses current evidence-based knowledge, including research findings, to guide practice.

▶ Incorporates evidence when initiating changes in nursing practice.

▶ Participates, as appropriate to educational level and position, in the formulation of evidence-based practice through research.

▶ Promotes ethical principles of research in practice and the healthcare setting.

▶ Appraises nursing research for optimal application in practice and the healthcare setting.

▶ Shares peer-reviewed research findings with colleagues to integrate knowledge into nursing practice.

Additional competencies for the graduate-level-prepared faith community nurse, including the APRN

In addition to the competencies of the faith community nurse, the graduate-level-prepared faith community nurse or advanced practice faith community nurse:

▶ Integrates research-based practice in all settings.

▶ Uses current healthcare research findings and other evidence to expand knowledge, skills, abilities, and judgment; to enhance role performance; and to increase knowledge of professional issues.

▶ Uses critical thinking skills to connect theory and research to practice.

- ▶ Integrates nursing research to improve quality in nursing practice.

- ▶ Recognizes the critical need for measuring research in the spiritual dimensions of diagnosis, interventions, and outcomes that improve health and wholeness for individuals, families, and communities.

- ▶ Contributes to nursing knowledge by conducting or synthesizing research and other evidence that discovers, examines, and evaluates current practice, knowledge, theories, criteria, and creative approaches to improve healthcare outcomes and integrating spiritual care and nursing care in a faith community.

- ▶ Designs strategies and tactics to meet the multifaceted and complex needs of healthcare consumers as well as population health programs.

- ▶ Leads the design and development of interprofessional processes to address the identified diagnoses, problems, or issues at both the individual level as well as population health level.

- ▶ Encourages other nurses to develop research skills.

- ▶ Designs innovative nursing practices to improve the health and well-being of individual and communities (populations).

- ▶ Performs rigorous critique of evidence derived from databases to generate meaningful evidence for nursing practice.

- ▶ Advocates for the ethical conduct of research and translational scholarship with particular attention to the protection of the healthcare consumer as a research participant.

- ▶ Promotes a climate of collaborative research and clinical inquiry.

- ▶ Disseminates research findings through activities such as presentations, publications, consultation, and journal clubs.

Standard 14. Quality of Practice

The faith community nurse contributes to quality nursing practice.

Competencies

The faith community nurse:

- Ensures that nursing practice is safe, effective, efficient, equitable, timely, and patient centered (IOM, 1999, 2001).
- Identifies barriers and opportunities to improve healthcare safety, effectiveness, efficiency, equitability, timeliness, and patient-centeredness.
- Recommends strategies to improve nursing quality.
- Uses creativity and innovation to enhance nursing care.
- Participates in quality improvement initiatives.
- Collects data to monitor the quality of nursing practice.
- Contributes in efforts to improve healthcare efficiency.
- Provides critical review and/or evaluation of policies, procedures, and guidelines to improve the quality of health care.
- Engages in formal and informal peer review processes.
- Collaborates with the interprofessional team to implement quality improvement plans and interventions.
- Documents nursing practice in a manner that supports quality and performance improvement initiatives.
- Achieves professional certification in faith community nursing.

Additional competencies for the graduate-level-prepared faith community nurse

In addition to the competencies for the faith community nurse, the graduate-level-prepared faith community nurse:

- Analyzes trends in healthcare quality data, including examination of cultural, spiritual, and religious influences and factors.
- Incorporates evidence into nursing practice to improve outcomes.

- Designs innovations to improve outcomes.
- Provides leadership in the design and implementation of quality improvement initiatives.
- Promotes a practice environment that supports evidence-based health care.
- Contributes to nursing and interprofessional knowledge through scientific inquiry.
- Encourages professional or specialty certification.
- Engages in development, implementation, evaluation, and/or revision of policies, procedures, and guidelines to improve healthcare quality.
- Uses data and information in system-level decision-making.
- Influences the organizational system to improve outcomes.

Additional competencies for the advanced practice faith community nurse

In addition to the competencies for the faith community nurse and graduate-level-prepared faith community nurse, the advanced practice faith community nurse:

- Engages in comparison evaluations of the effectiveness and efficacy of diagnostic tests, clinical procedures and therapies, and treatment plans, in partnership with healthcare consumers, to optimize health and healthcare quality.
- Designs quality improvement studies, research, initiatives, and programs to improve health outcomes in diverse settings.
- Applies knowledge obtained from advanced preparation, as well as current research and evidence-based information, to clinical decision-making at the point of care to achieve optimal health outcomes.
- Uses available benchmarks as a means to evaluate practice at the individual, departmental, or organizational level.

Standard 15. Professional Practice Evaluation

The faith community nurse evaluates one's own and others' nursing practice.

Competencies

The faith community nurse:

▶ Engages in self-reflection and self-evaluation of nursing practice on a regular basis, identifying areas of strength as well as areas in which professional and spiritual growth would be beneficial.

▶ Adheres to the guidance about professional practice as specified in the *Nursing: Scope and Standards of Practice* and the *Code of Ethics for Nurses with Interpretive Statements*.

▶ Ensures that nursing practice is consistent with regulatory requirements pertaining to licensure, relevant statutes, rules, and regulations.

▶ Uses organizational policies and procedures to guide professional practice.

▶ Influences organizational policies and procedures to promote inter-professional evidence-based practice.

▶ Provides evidence for practice decisions and actions as part of the formal and informal evaluation processes.

▶ Seeks formal and informal feedback regarding one's own practice from healthcare consumers, peers, colleagues, supervisors, faith leaders, and others.

▶ Provides peers and others with formal and informal constructive feedback regarding their practice or role performance.

▶ Takes action to achieve goals identified during the evaluation process.

Standard 16. Resource Utilization

The faith community nurse utilizes appropriate resources to plan, provide, and sustain evidence-based nursing services that are safe, effective, and fiscally responsible.

Competencies

The faith community nurse:

▶ Assesses healthcare consumer care needs and resources available to achieve desired outcomes.

▶ Assists the healthcare consumer in factoring costs, risks, and benefits in decisions about treatment and care.

▶ Assists the healthcare consumer in identifying and securing appropriate services to address health and spiritually related needs across the healthcare continuum.

▶ Delegates in accordance with applicable legal and policy parameters.

▶ Identifies impact of resource allocation on the potential for harm, complexity of the task, and desired outcomes.

▶ Advocates for resources that support and enhance nursing practice.

▶ Integrates telehealth and mobile health technologies into practice to promote positive interactions between healthcare consumers and care providers.

▶ Uses organizational and community resources to implement interprofessional plans.

▶ Addresses discriminatory healthcare practices and the impact on resource allocation.

Additional competencies for the graduate-level-prepared faith community nurse

In addition to the competencies of the faith community nurse, the graduate-level-prepared faith community nurse:

▶ Designs innovative solutions to use resources effectively and maintain quality.

▶ Creates evaluation strategies that address cost effectiveness, cost–benefit, and efficiency factors associated with nursing practice.

- ▶ Assumes complex and advanced leadership roles to initiate and guide change.
- ▶ Uses organizational and community resources to formulate interprofessional plans of care.

Additional competencies for the advanced practice faith community nurse

In addition to the competencies of the faith community nurse and graduate-level-prepared faith community nurse, the advanced practice faith community nurse:

- ▶ Engages organizational and community resources to formulate and implement interprofessional plans.

Standard 17. Environmental Health

The faith community nurse practices in an environmentally safe and healthy manner.

Competencies

The faith community nurse:

- ► Promotes a safe and healthy community professional practice environment.
- ► Uses environmental health concepts in practice.
- ► Assesses the environment to identify risk factors.
- ► Reduces environmental health risks to self, colleagues, and health-care consumers, and community.
- ► Communicates information about environmental health risks and exposure reduction strategies.
- ► Participates in developing social, political, and economic strategies to promote healthy communities and practice environments.
- ► Advocates for environmental health and social justice, including a commitment to the health of vulnerable populations.
- ► Advocates for the safe, judicious, and appropriate use and disposal of products in health care.
- ► Incorporates technologies to promote safe practice environments.
- ► Uses products or treatments consistent with evidence-based practice to reduce environmental threats.

Additional competencies for the graduate-level-prepared faith community nurse, including the APRN

In addition to the competencies of the faith community nurse, the graduate-level-prepared faith community nurse:

▶ Analyzes the impact of social, political, and economic influences on the global environment and human health experience.

▶ Creates partnerships that promote sustainable global environmental health policies and conditions that focus on prevention of hazards to people and the natural environment (ANA, 2007).

▶ Identifies patterns of comorbidities among family and community members suggesting environmental etiologies.

Glossary

Acculturation. The process by which an individual or group from one culture learns how to take on many of the behaviors, values, and ways of living of another culture. Few cultures become 100% acculturated to another cultural way of life. Cultures tend to be selective in what they choose to change and retain (Leininger, 1995, pp. 72–73).

Advanced practice registered nurse (APRN). A registered nurse who has completed an accredited graduate-level education program preparing her or him for the role of certified nurse practitioner, certified registered nurse anesthetist, certified nurse midwife, or clinical nurse specialist; has passed a national certification examination that measures the APRN role and population-focused competencies; maintains continued competence as evidenced by recertification; and is licensed to practice as an APRN (ANA, 2015b, p. 85).

Advocacy. The act or process of pleading for, supporting, or recommending a cause or course of action. Advocacy may be for persons (whether as an individual, group, population, or society) or for an issue, such as potable water or global health (ANA, 2015a, p. 41).

Assessment. A systematic, dynamic process by which a faith community registered nurse, through interaction with the healthcare consumer, family, groups, communities, populations, spiritual leaders, and healthcare providers, collects and analyzes data. In addition to spiritual dimensions, assessment by the faith community registered nurse may include the following dimensions: physical, psychological, sociocultural, cognitive, functional abilities, developmental, economic, environmental, and lifestyle (ANA, 2015b, p. 85).

Autonomy. The capacity of a nurse to determine her or his own actions through independent choice, including demonstration of competence, within the full scope of nursing practice (ANA, 2015b, p. 85).

Behavioral health. A branch of interdisciplinary health that focuses on the reciprocal relationship between the holistic view of human behavior and the well-being of the body as a whole entity (https://medanth.wikispaces.com/Behavioral+Health).

Caregiver. A person who provides direct care for another, such as a child, dependent adult, the disabled, spiritually distressed, or the chronically ill (ANA, 2015b, p. 85).

Caring. The moral ideal of nursing consisting of human-to-human attempts to protect, enhance, and preserve humanity and human dignity, integrity, and wholeness by assisting a person to find meaning in illness, suffering, pain, and existence (Watson, 2012).

Certification. A process by which a nongovernmental agency or association certifies that an individual licensed to practice a profession has met certain predetermined standards specified by that profession for specialty practice. Its purpose is to assure various publics that an individual has mastered a body of knowledge and acquired skills in a particular specialty (ANA, 1979, p. 67).

Code of ethics (nursing). A list of provisions that makes explicit the primary goals, values, and obligations of the nursing profession and expresses its values, duties, and commitments to the society of which it is a part. In the United States, nurses abide by and adhere to *Code of Ethics for Nurses with Interpretive Statements* (ANA, 2015b, p. 86).

Collaboration. A professional healthcare partnership grounded in a reciprocal and respectful recognition and acceptance of each partner's unique expertise, power, and sphere of influence and responsibilities; the commonality of goals; the mutual safeguarding of the legitimate interest of each party; and the advantages of such a relationship (ANA, 2015b, p. 86).

Competency. An expected and measurable level of nursing performance that integrates knowledge, skills, abilities, and judgment and that is based on established scientific knowledge and expectations for nursing practice (ANA, 2015b, p. 86).

Confidentiality. A right to have one's private, intimate, or secret information kept undisclosed to a third party unless permission is granted for disclosure (ANA, 2015a, p. 42).

Continuity of care. An interdisciplinary process that includes healthcare consumers, families, significant others, and appropriate members of a faith community in the development of a coordinated plan of care. This process facilitates the healthcare consumer's transition between settings and healthcare providers, based on changing needs and available resources (ANA, 2015b, p. 86).

Cultural knowledge. The concepts and language of an ethnic or social group used to describe their health-related values, beliefs, and traditional practices, as well as the etiologies of their conditions, preferred treatments, and any contra-indications for treatments or pharmacological interventions. Historical events, such as war-related migration, oppression, and structural discrimination are also included, when relevant (ANA, 2015b, p. 86).

Cultural skills. The integration of cultural knowledge and expertise into prac-tice when assessing, communicating with, and providing care for members of a racial, ethnic or social group (ANA, 2015b, p. 86).

Delegation. The transfer of responsibility for the performance of a task from one individual to another while retaining accountability for the outcome. Example: The registered nurse, in delegating a task to an assistive individual, transfers the responsibility for the performance of the task but retains profes-sional accountability for the overall care (ANA, 2015b, p. 86).

Diagnosis. A clinical judgment about the healthcare consumer's response to actual, perceived, or potential health concerns or needs. The diagnosis provides the basis for determining a plan to achieve desired outcomes, to establish priorities, and to develop a plan of action with the healthcare consumer. Faith community registered nurses utilize nursing diagnoses or medical diagnoses depending on their education, clinical preparation, and legal authority (ANA, 2015b, p. 86).

Disease. A biological or psychosocial disorder of structure or function in a healthcare consumer, especially a disorder that produces specific signs or symptoms or that affects a specific part of the body, mind, or spirit.

Documentation. The recording of the assessment, plan of care, interventions, and evaluation of outcomes in a retrievable format that is confidential and secure for the healthcare consumer to facilitate continuity in meeting desired health outcomes.

Ecosystem. A system, or a group of interconnected elements, formed by the interaction of a community of organisms with their environment (ANA, 2015b, p. 87).

Environment. The surrounding habitat, context, milieu, conditions, and atmo-sphere in which all living systems participate and interact. It includes the phys-ical habitat as well as cultural, psychological, social, religious, and historical influences. It includes both the external physical space as well as an individual's internal physical, mental, emotional, social, and spiritual experience (ANA/AHNA, 2013).

Environmental health. Aspects of human health, including quality of life, that are determined by physical, chemical, biological, social, and psychological influences in the environment. It also refers to the theory and practice of assessing, correcting, controlling, and preventing those factors in the environment that can potentially adversely affect the health of present and future generations (ANA, 2015b, p. 87).

Evaluation. The process of determining the progress toward attainment of expected outcomes, including the effectiveness of care (ANA, 2015b, p. 87).

Evidence-based practice (EBP). A lifelong problem-solving approach that integrates the best evidence from well-designed research studies and evidence-based theories; clinical expertise and evidence from assessment of the health consumer's history and condition, as well as healthcare resources; and patient, family, group, community, and population preferences and values. When EBP is delivered in a context of caring, as well as an ecosystem or environment that supports it, the best clinical decisions are made to yield positive healthcare consumer outcomes (Melnyk, Gallagher-Ford, Long, & Fineout-Overholt, 2014).

Expected outcomes. End results that are measurable, desirable, and observable and translate into observable behaviors (ANA, 2015b, p. 87).

Faith community. An organization of groups, families, and individuals who share common values, beliefs, religious doctrine, and faith practices that influence their lives, generally in the setting of a church, synagogue, temple, mosque or faith-based agency, and that functions as a healthcare consumer system, providing a setting for faith community nursing.

Faith community nurse (FCN). A registered professional nurse who is actively licensed in a given state and who serves as a member of the staff of a faith community. The FCN promotes health as wholeness of the faith community, its groups, families, and individual members through the practice of nursing as defined by that state's nurse practice act in the jurisdiction in which the FCN practices and the standards of practice set forth in this document.

Faith community nursing. The specialized practice of professional nursing focusing on the intentional care of the spirit as the foundation of the practice. The delivery of care and relationship established promotes whole-person health and prevention or minimization of illness within the context of a faith community and the wider community.

Faith group. A specific denomination or sect within a faith tradition.

Family. Family of origin or significant others as identified by a healthcare consumer, who may refer to some or all of the members of a faith community as part of their family (ANA, 2015b, p. 87).

Graduate-level-prepared registered nurse. A registered nurse prepared at the master's or doctoral educational level who has advanced knowledge, skills, abilities, and judgment; functions in an advanced level as designated by elements of his or her position; and is not required to have additional regulatory oversight (ANA, 2015b, p. 87).

Group. A number of people sharing something in common, such as an interest, activity, or spiritual beliefs and practices.

Healing. The process of integrating the body, mind, and spirit to bring about wholeness, health, and a sense of spiritual well-being, although the healthcare consumer's disease may not be cured.

Health. The experience of wholeness, salvation, or shalom. The integration of the spiritual, physical, psychological, emotional, and social aspects of the healthcare consumer to create a sense of harmony with self, others, the environment, and a higher power. Health may be experienced in the presence or absence of disease or injury.

Health ministry. The promotion of health and healing as part of the mission and service of a faith community to its members and the community it serves.

Health promotion. Activities and interventions that healthcare consumers undertake to achieve desired health outcomes. Health promotion outcomes may be primary (the prevention of disease and injury), secondary (the early detection and appropriate intervention in illness or brokenness), or tertiary (the promotion of wholeness and sense of well-being when curing may not occur).

Healthcare consumer. The person, client, family, group, community, or population who is the focus of attention and to whom the registered nurse is providing services as sanctioned by the state regulatory bodies. The term *healthcare consumer* is used to provide consistency and brevity, bearing in mind that other terms, such as *client, individual, family, groups, community,* or *population*, might be better choices in some instances.

- When the healthcare consumer is an individual, the focus is on the health state, problems, or needs of the individual.
- When the healthcare consumer is a family or group, the focus is on the health of the unit as a whole or the reciprocal effects of the individual's health on the other members of the unit.

- When the healthcare consumer is a community or population, the focus is on personal and environmental health and the health risks of the community or population.

Healthcare providers. Individuals with special expertise who provide healthcare services or assistance to healthcare consumers. They may include nurses, physicians, spiritual leaders, psychologists, social workers, nutritionists/dietitians, and various therapists (ANA, 2015b, p. 88).

Holistic care. The integration of body–mind–emotion–spirit–sexual–cultural–social–energetic–environmental principles and modalities to promote health, increase well-being, and actualize human potential (ANA, 2015b, p. 88).

Illness. The subjective experience of discomfort, brokenness; the disintegration of body, mind, spirit; disharmony with others, the environment, or a higher power. Not synonymous with disease (ANA, 2015b, p. 88).

Implementation. Activities such as teaching, monitoring, providing, praying, leading meditation, counseling, delegating, and coordinating. Carrying out of a plan of action in a spiritual, caring relationship that provides the information, skills, motivation, spiritual, or faith tradition rituals and resources necessary to empower the healthcare consumer to achieve desired health outcomes.

Information. Data that are interpreted, organized, or structured (ANA, 2015b, p. 88).

Intentional care of the spirit. The delivery of care that promotes whole-person-centered well-being, establishes a therapeutic relationship, with caring as a sacred practice, and focuses on the relationship between faith and health.

Interprofessional. Reliant on overlapping knowledge, skills, and abilities of each team member and discipline, resulting in synergistic effects where outcomes are enhanced and more comprehensive than the simple aggregation of any team member's individual efforts (ANA, 2015b, p. 88).

Interprofessional collaboration. Integrated enactment of knowledge, skills, and values and attitudes that define working together across the professions, with other healthcare workers, and with patients, along with families and communities, as appropriate to improve health outcomes (Interprofessional Education Collaborative Expert Panel, 2011).

Mental health. A state of well-being in which every individual realizes his or her own potential, can cope with the normal stresses of life, can work productively and fruitfully, and is able to make a contribution to her or his community (World Health Organization, 2001).

Moral agent. An individual who is morally obligated or capable of acting with reference to right and wrong. (Moral agent, n.d.)

Nursing. The protection, promotion, and optimization of health and abilities; prevention of illness and injury; facilitation of healing; alleviation of suffering through the diagnosis and treatment of human response; and advocacy in the care of individuals, families, groups, communities, and populations (ANA, 2015b, p. 88).

Nursing practice. The collective professional activities of nurses characterized by the interrelations of human responses, theory application, nursing actions, and outcomes (ANA, 2015b, p. 88).

Nursing process. A critical thinking model used by nurses that is represented as the integration of the singular, concurrent actions of these six components: assessment, diagnosis, identification of outcomes, planning, implementation, and evaluation (ANA, 2015b, p. 88).

Patient. See *Healthcare consumer*.

Peer review. A collegial, systematic, and periodic process by which faith community nurses are held accountable for their practice and that fosters the refinement of one's knowledge, skills, and decision-making at all levels and in all areas of practice.

Plan. A comprehensive outline of the components that need to be completed to attain mutually identified and expected healthcare consumer outcomes.

Population. The number or body of inhabitants in a place belonging to a specific social, cultural, socioeconomic, ethnic, or racial group. A group of individual persons, objects, or items from which samples are taken for statistical measurement.

Population health. The health outcomes of a group of individuals, including the distribution of such outcomes within the group, and we argue that the field of population health includes health outcomes, patterns of health determinants, and policies and interventions that link these two (National Center for Biotechnology Information, 2003).

Quality of care. The degree to which health services for healthcare consumers, families, groups, communities, or populations increase the likelihood of desired outcomes and are consistent with current professional knowledge (ANA, 2015b, p. 89).

Registered nurse (RN). An individual registered or licensed by a state, commonwealth, territory, government, or other regulatory body to practice as a registered nurse (ANA, 2015b, p. 89).

Restorative practices. Nursing interventions that mitigate the impact of illness or disease.

Scope of nursing practice. The description of the *who, what, where, when, why,* and *how* of nursing practice that addresses the range of nursing practice activities common to all registered nurses. When considered in conjunction with the *Standards of Professional Nursing Practice* and the *Code of Ethics for Nurses,* comprehensively describes the competent level of nursing common to all registered nurses (ANA, 2015b, p. 89).

Self-care. Actions an individual, family, group, or faith community takes to attain desired holistic health outcomes when they possess the requisite knowledge, skills, ability, resources, motivation, encouragement, and support.

Social determinants of health. Conditions in the environments in which people are born, live, learn, work, play, worship, and age that affect a wide range of health, functioning, and quality-of-life outcomes and risks (Healthy People 2020, 2014).

Social justice. A form of justice that engages in social criticism and social change. Its focus is the analysis, critique, and change of social structures, policies, laws, customs, power, and privilege that disadvantage or harm vulnerable social groups through marginalization, exclusion, exploitation, and voicelessness. Among its ends are a more equitable distribution of social and economic benefits and burdens; greater personal, social, and political dignity; and a deeper moral vision for society. It may refer to a theory, process, or end (ANA, 2015a, p. 46).

Spiritual care. The practical expression of presence, guidance, and interventions, individual or communal, to support, nurture, or encourage an individual's or group's ability to achieve wholeness; health; personal, spiritual, religious, and social well-being; integration of body, mind, and spirit; and a sense of connection to self, others, and a higher power.

Spiritual leader. An individual recognized and authorized by a faith community, such as a clergyperson (pastor, priest, rabbi, and shaman), chaplain, or lay minister, who guides and inspires others in the study and nurture of their spiritual beliefs and application of spiritual practices.

Stakeholder. A person, group or organization that has interest or concern in an organization. Stakeholders can affect or be affected by the organization's actions, objectives and policies.

Standard. An authoritative statement defined and promoted by the profession by which the quality of practice, service, or education can be evaluated (ANA, 2015b, p. 89).

Standards of Practice. Standards that describe a competent level of nursing care as demonstrated by the nursing process. *See also* Nursing process (ANA, 2015b, p. 89).

Standards of Professional Nursing Practice. Authoritative statements of the duties that all registered nurses, regardless of role, population, or specialty, are expected to perform competently (ANA, 2015b, p. 89).

Standards of Professional Performance. Standards that describe a competent level of behavior in the professional role (ANA, 2015b, p. 89).

Supportive practices. Nursing interventions that are oriented toward modification of relationships or the environment to support health.

Transitional care. Actions of faith community nurses and other healthcare providers designed to ensure the coordination and continuity of health care for healthcare consumers during movement between hospitals, subacute and postacute nursing facilities, the healthcare consumer's home, primary and specialty care offices, and long-term care facilities as their condition and care needs change during the course of a chronic or acute illness.

Volunteer. A volunteer is a person who offers a service freely without expectation of payment. In the context of health ministry, the volunteer is one who offers services within the faith community as differentiated from the faith community nurse serving as unpaid staff.

Well-being. An individual's perception of her or his own wholistic health.

Wellness. Integrated, congruent functioning aimed toward reaching one's highest potential (ANA/AHNA, 2013).

Whole-person health. Integration of an individual's emotional, intellectual, physical, social, spiritual, and vocational dimensions into positive beliefs and meaningful activities that enhance human functioning and quality of life. It includes an openness to change, capacity to deal with stress, and a personal view of self-worth.

Wholistic. Based on an understanding that a healthcare consumer is an interconnected unity and that physical, mental, social, environmental, and spiritual factors need to be included in any interventions. The whole system, whether referring to a human being or a faith community, is greater than the sum of its parts. Term may be used in place of *holistic* when referring to the type of care provided by a faith community nurse.

Worldview. The way people look out at their universe and form a picture or value about their lives and the world around them (Leininger, 1995, p. 105). "Worldview includes one's relationship with nature, moral and ethical reasoning, social relationships, and magico-religious beliefs" (Purnell & Paulanka, 1998, p. 3), among others (ANA, 2015b, p. 89).

References and Bibliography

Agency for Healthcare Research and Quality. (2014). Improve hospital-based transitional care processes for Medicaid patients. Retrieved from http://www.ahrq.gov/professionals/systems /hospital/medicaidreadmitguide/medread-sec4.html

American Association of Colleges of Nursing (AACN). (2000). *AACN position statement on the Baccalaureate Degree in Nursing as Minimal Preparation for Professional Practice.* Washington, DC: Author.

American Association of Colleges of Nursing. (2016). *Advancing healthcare transformation: A new era for academic nursing.* Washington, DC: Author.

American Nurses Association (ANA). (1979). *The study of credentialing in nursing: A new approach.* Kansas City, MO: American Nurses Association, p. 67.

American Nurses Association (ANA). (2000). *Scope and standards of public health nursing practice.* Silver Spring, MD: Nursebooks.org.

American Nurses Association (ANA). (2013). 2013 Membership assembly environmental scan summary. Retrieved from http://nursingworld.org/HomepageCategory/NursingInsider /Archive-1/2013-NI/June-2013-NI/ANA-Holds-Inaugural-Membership-Assembly.html

American Nurses Association (ANA). (2014). *Professional role competence (Position Statement).* Silver Spring, MD: Author.

American Nurses Association (ANA). (2015a). *Code of ethics for nurses with interpretive statements.* Silver Spring, MD: Nursesbooks.org.

American Nurses Association (ANA). (2015b). *Nursing: Scope and standards of practice* (3rd ed.). Silver Spring, MD: Nursebooks.org.

American Nurses Association (ANA). (2015c). *Guide to nursing's social policy statement: Understanding the profession from social contract to social covenant.* Silver Spring, MD: Nursebooks.org.

American Nurses Association (ANA). (2016). Higher education: Learning what it means to provide spiritual care. *The American Nurse.* Retrieved from http://www.theamericannurse .org/2016/11/01/higher-education/.

American Nurses Association (ANA). (2017). Official ANA position statements. Retrieved from http://nursingworld.org/MainMenuCategories/Policy-Advocacy/Positions-and-Resolutions /ANAPositionStatements

American Nurses Association and American Holistic Nurses Association (ANA/AHNA). (2013). *Holistic nursing: Scope & standards of practice* (2nd ed.). Silver Spring, MD: Nursebooks.org.

American Psychiatric Association. (2016). Patients' spirituality useful to healing process. Retrieved from http://psychnews.psychiatryonline.org/doi/full/10.1176/pn.41.16.0018

Anaebere, A. K., & Delilly, C. R. (2012). Faith community nursing: Supporting mental health during life transitions. *Issues in Mental Health Nursing, 33,* 337–339.

APRN Joint Dialogue Group. 2008. *Consensus Model for APRN Regulation: Licensure, accreditation, certification, and education*. Retrieved from http://www.nursingworld.org/ConsensusModelforAPRN

Asomugha, C. N., Derose, K., & Lurie, N. (2011). Faith-based organizations, science, and the pursuit of health. *Journal of Health Care for the Poor and Underserved, 22*, 50–55. doi: 10.1353/hpu.2011.0008. Retrieved March 21, 2017, from https://www.ncbi.nlm.nih.gov/pmc/articles/PMC3074611/

Bachrach, C., & Thomas, Y. (2016, June). Training nurses in population health science: What, why, how? Presentation at the 133rd meeting of the National Advisory Council for Nurse Education and Practice, Rockville, MD.

Balboni, M. J., Sullivan, A., Enzinger, A. C., Epstein-Peterson, Z. D., Tseng, Y. D., Mitchell, C., & Balboni, T. A. (2014). Nurse and physician barriers to spiritual care provision at the end of life. *Journal of Pain and Symptom Management, 48*(3), 400–410.

Balint, K. A. & George, N. M. (2015). Faith community nursing scope of practice: extending access to healthcare. *Journal of Christian Nursing, 32*(1), 34–40.

Beauchamp, T., & Childress, J. (2009). *Principles of biomedical ethics*. Oxford University Press.

Brown, A., Coppola, P., Giacona, M., Petriches, A., & Stockwell, M. A. (2009). Faith community nursing demonstrates good stewardship of community benefit dollars through cost savings and cost avoidance. *Family & Community Health, 32*(4), 330–338. doi: 10.1097/FCH.0b013e3181b91f93.

Campinha-Bacote, J. (2011). Coming to know cultural competence: An evolutionary process. *International Journal For Human Caring, 15*(3), 42–48.

Canadian Center for Occupational Health and Safety (CCOHS). (2016). Violence in the Workplace. Retrieved from http://www.ccohs.ca/oshanswers/psychosocial/violence.html

Center for Nursing Classification and Clinical Effectiveness. (n.d.) Retrieved from https://nursing.uiowa.edu/center-for-nursing-classification-and-clinical-effectiveness

Chase-Ziolek, M. (2017). The gift of spiritual direction: Listening well, digging deep, and letting go. *Church Health Reader*. Memphis, TN: Church Health Center. Retrieved March 20, 2017, from http://chreader.org/the-gift-of-spiritual-direction/

Corley, M. C. (2002). Nurse moral distress: A proposed theory and research agenda. *Nursing Ethics, 9*(6), 636–650.

Donahue, M. P. (1996). *Nursing—The finest art: An illustrated history* (2nd ed.). St. Louis, MO: Mosby.

Dunn, H. L. (1959). High-level wellness for man and society. *Journal of Public Health, 49*(6), 786–792.

Health Ministries Association (HMA). (2017). The diary of a faith community nurse [HMA website]. Retrieved March 8, 2017, from http://hmassoc.org/the-diary-of-a-faith-community-nurse/

Health Ministries Association (HMA) and American Nurses Association (ANA). (2012). *Faith community nursing: Scope and standards practice* (2nd ed.). Silver Spring, MD: Nursesbooks.org.

Health Resources Services Administration. (2016). What is telehealth? How is telehealth different from telemedicine? Retrieved from https://www.healthit.gov/providers-professionals/faqs/what-telehealth-how-telehealth-different-telemedicine

Healthy People 2020. (2014). *Social determinants of health*. Retrieved from https://www.healthypeople.gov/2020/topics-objectives/topic/social-determinants-of-health

Hickman, J. (2006). *Faith community nursing*. Philadelphia, PA: Lippincott, Williams, & Wilkins.

Hickman, J. (2011). *Fast facts for the faith community nurse: Implementing FCN/parish nursing in a nutshell.* New York, NY: Springer, pp. 29–35.

Institute of Medicine (IOM). (1999). *To err is human: Building a safer health system.* Washington, DC: National Academies Press.

Institute of Medicine (IOM). (2001). *Crossing the quality chasm: A new health system for the 21st century.* Washington, DC: National Academies Press.

Institute of Medicine (IOM). (2010). *The future of nursing: Leading change, advancing health.* Washington, DC: National Academies Press.

International Parish Nurse Resource Center. (2014). *Foundations of faith community nursing curriculum.* Memphis TN: Church Health Center.

Interprofessional Education Collaborative Expert Panel (IECEP). (2011). *Core competencies for interprofessional collaborative practice: Report of an expert panel.* Washington, DC: Interprofessional Education Collaborative. Also available online: http://www.aacn.nche.edu/education-resources/ipecreport.pdf

Jameton, A. (1984). *Nursing practice: The ethical issues.* Englewood Cliffs, NJ: Prentice-Hall.

Jonsen, A., Siegler, M., & Winslade, W. (2006). *Clinical ethics: A practical approach to ethical decisions in clinical medicine* (6th ed.). New York: McGraw-Hill.

Koenig, H. (2012). Religion, spirituality, and health: The research and clinical implications. *ISRN Psychiatry, 2012,* 278730. doi: 10.5402/2012/278730

Leddy, S. K. (2006). *Health promotion: Mobilizing strengths to enhance health, wellness, and well-being* (1st ed.). Philadelphia: FA Davis.

Leininger, M. (1995). *Transcultural nursing. Concepts, theories, research & practices* (2nd ed.). New York: McGraw-Hill, Inc.

Leininger, M., & McFarland, M. (2002). *Transcultural nursing. Concepts, theories, research & practices (3rd ed.).* New York: McGraw-Hill, Inc.

Martin, K. S. & Monsen, K. A. (2016).The omaha system: Solving the clinical data-information puzzle. Retrieved March 15, 2017, from http://omahasystem.org/overview.html

Melnyk, B., Gallagher-Ford, L., Long, L., & Fineout-Overholt, E. (2014). The establishment of evidence-based practice competencies for practicing registered nurses and advanced practice nurses in real-world clinical settings: Proficiencies to improve healthcare quality, reliability, patient outcomes, and costs. *Worldviews Evidence-Based Nursing, 11,* 5–15. doi: 10.1111/wvn.12021

Modern Health Care. (2014). Retrieved from http://www.modernhealthcare.com/article/20140308/MAGAZINE/303089979

Moral agent. (n.d.) *Segen's Medical Dictionary.* (2011). Retrieved June 14 2017 from http://medical-dictionary.thefreedictionary.com/moral+agent

NANDA International (NANDA). (2012). *Nursing diagnoses: Definitions and classification 2012–2014.* Retrieved from www.wiley.com/wiley-blackwell

NANDA International. (n.d.) Retrieved from http://www.nanda.org/

National Alliance on Mental Illness. (2016). NAMI Faith Net: How to be inclusive and welcoming. Retrieved from https://www.nami.org/Get-Involved/NAMI-FaithNet/How-to-Be-Inclusive-and-Welcoming

National Center for Biotechnology Information. National Institutes for Health (NCBI). (2003). Retrieved from http://www.ncbi.nlm.nih.gov/pmc/articles/PMC1447747).

Naylor, M. D., Bowles, K. H., McCauley, K. M., MacCoy, M. C., Maislin, G., Pauly, M. V., & Krakauer. R. (2011). High-value transitional care: Translation of research into practice. *Journal of Evaluation in Clinical Practice, −19*(5), 727–733. doi: 10.1111/j.1365-2753.2011.01659.x.

Newman, M. (1995). *A developing discipline: Selected works of Margaret Newman*. New York: National League for Nursing.

Pew Research Center (PEW). (2012). Retrieved from http://www.pewinternet.org/fact-sheets/health-fact-sheet/

Puchalski, C. (2012). Spirituality in the cancer trajectory. *Annals of Oncology, 32*(3), 49–55.

Purnell, L. D., & Paulanka, B. J. (1998). *Transcultural health care: A culturally competent approach*. Philadelphia, PA: F. A. Davis, Co.

Reilly, J., Hovarter, R., Mrochek, T., Mittelstadt-Lock, K., Schmitz, S., Nett, S., …, Behm, L. (2011). Spread the word, not germs: A toolkit for faith communities. *Journal of Christian Nursing, 28*(4), 205–211.

Robert Wood Johnson (RWJ). (2010). Rural nursing facing unique workforce challenges. Retrieved January 10, 2017, from http://www.rwjf.org/en/library/articles-and-news/2010/09/rural-nursing-facing-unique-workforce-challenges.html

Roy, C. (1976). *Introduction to nursing: An adaptation model*. Burlington, MA: Jones & Bartlett.

Rushton, C., Schoonover-Shoffner, K., & Kennedy, M. (2017). A collaborative state of the science initiative: Transforming moral distress into moral resilience in nursing. *AJN, American Journal of Nursing, 117*(2), S2–S6. Retrieved from at http://journals.lww.com/ajnonline/toc/2017/02001

Saba, V. (2017) Clinical Care Classification System. Retrieved March 15, 2017, from https://www.sabacare.com/framework/.

Schroepfer, C. (2016). A renewed look at faith community nursing. *MedSurg Nursing, 25*(1), 62–66. Retrieved March 8, 2017, from http://www.pnmny.org/articles/ARenewedLookatFaithCommunityNursingMSN%20J-F16.pdf

Sharma, R. K., Astrow, A. B., Texeira, K., & Sulmasy, D. P. (2012). The Spiritual Needs Assessment for Patients (SNAP): Development and validation of a comprehensive instrument to assess unmet spiritual needs. *Journal of Pain and Symptom Management, 44*(1), 44–51.

Skemp, E., Dreher, M., & Lehmann, S. (2016). *Healthy places healthy people: A handbook for culturally informed community nursing practice, third edition*. Indianapolis, IN: Sigma Theta Tau International Honor Society of Nursing.

Smucker, C. (2008). *Faith Community Nursing: Developing a Quality Practice*. Silver Spring, MD: Nursebooks.org.

Solari-Twadell, P., & Hackbarth, D. (2010). Evidence for a new paradigm of the ministry of parish nursing practice using the nursing intervention classification system. *Nursing Outlook, 58*(2), 69–75. doi:10.1016/j.outlook.2009.09.003

Stolte, K. M. (1996). *Wellness nursing diagnosis for health promotion*. Philadelphia, PA: Lippincott, Williams, & Wilkins, p. 304.

Tay, L., Tan, K., Diener, E., & Gonzalez, E. (2013). Social Relations, health behaviors, and health outcomes a survey and synthesis. *Applied Psychology: Health and Well-Being*. Retrieved March 21, 2017, from http://www.rwjf.org/en/library/research/2013/03/social-relations-health-behaviors-and-health-outcomes.html

U.S. Census. (2016). Retrieved from https://www.census.gov/newsroom/press-releases/2016/cb16-210.html

Watson, J. (1985). *Nursing: Human science and human care: A theory of nursing*. Norwalk, CT: Appleton-Century-Crofts.

Watson, J. (2012). *Human caring science: A theory of nursing* (2nd ed.). Sudbury, MA: Jones and Bartlett Learning.

Westberg, G., & McNamara, J. (1990). *The parish nurse: Providing a minister of health for your congregation*. Minneapolis, MN: Augsburg Fortress.

Williams, J. A., Meltzer, D., Arora, V., Chung, G., & Curlin, F. A. (2011). Attention to inpatients' religious and spiritual concerns: predictors and association with patient satisfaction. *General Internal Medicine, 26*(11), 1265–1171. doi: 10.1007/s11606-011-1781-y.

World Health Organization. (2001). *Strengthening mental health promotion.* Geneva, Switzerland: World Health Organization (Fact Sheet No. 220).

Yeaworth, R. C., & Sailors, R. (2014). Faith community nursing: Real care, real cost savings. *Journal of Christian Nursing, 31*(3): 178–183.

Appendix A
Faith Community Nursing: *Scope and Standards of Practice, Second Edition (2012)*

FPO

AMERICAN NURSES ASSOCIATION

HEALTH

MINISTRIES
ASSOCIATION • INC.

Scope AND
Standards
OF PRACTICE

Faith
Community
Nursing

2ND EDITION

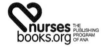

American Nurses Association
Silver Spring, Maryland
2012

Library of Congress Cataloging-in-Publication Data

Faith community nursing : scope and standards of practice. — 2nd ed.
p. ; cm.

Rev. ed. of: Faith community nursing / Health Ministries Association. 2005.

Includes bibliographical references and index.

Summary: "Delineates the practice of faith community nurses, which integrates the health and care of body, mind, and spirit in the context of a faith community, its professional roles, activities, expected accountabilities and competency levels per RN knowledge, skills, abilities, and judgment, education, professional development, and the specialty's history/legacy and trends"—Provided by publisher.

ISBN 978-1-55810-429-7—ISBN 978-1-55810-430-3 (pdf eBook)—ISBN 978-1-55810-433-4 (pdf eBook for site licenses)—ISBN 978-1-55810-431-0 (eBook, Mobipocket format)

I. American Nurses Association. II. Health Ministries Association. Faith community nursing. [DNLM: 1. Community Health Nursing—standards—Practice Guideline. 2. Spirituality—Practice Guideline. 3. Holistic Nursing--standards—Practice Guideline. 4. Nursing Process—standards—Practice Guideline. WY 87]

610.73'43—dc23

2011047488

Health Ministries Association (HMA) and American Nurses Association (ANA) are national professional associations. This joint HMA–ANA publication (*Faith Community Nursing: Scope and Standards of Practice, Second Edition*) reflects the thinking of the faith community nursing specialty on various issues and should be reviewed in conjunction with state board of nursing policies and practices. State law, rules, and regulations govern the practice of nursing, while *Faith Community Nursing: Scope and Standards of Practice, Second Edition* guides faith community nurses in the application of their professional skills and responsibilities.

ISBN-13: 978-1-55810-429-7   SAN: 851-3481   5K   01/2012

First printing: January 2012

Appendix A. *Faith Community Nursing: Scope and Standards of Practice, Second Edition (2012)*

Contents

Contributors

Faith Community Nursing Scope and Standards of Practice Work Group

Alyson J. Breisch, MSN, RN, FCN
Proprietor, Breisch Health Education, PLLC, Durham, North Carolina; Chair, Health Ministries Association FCN Standards Work Group, 2011
Ms. Breisch has more than 40 years experience in nursing administration, academic education, and advanced practice nursing as a clinical nurse specialist and adult nurse practitioner. She directed the graduate degree program in Health and Nursing Ministries of Duke Divinity School and Duke University School of Nursing and developed a continuing education curriculum for faith community nursing. She has been a faith community nurse for 12 years and a Commissioned Minister of Congregational Health for 5 years. Ms. Breisch is active in several professional nursing organizations. She is Director of Practice and Education on the Board of Directors of Health Ministries Association.

Jean Bokinskie, PhD, RN, FCN
Associate Professor of Nursing and Director of the Parish Nurse Ministry Program, Concordia College, Moorhead, Minnesota
Dr. Bokinskie has taught in nursing education for more than 20 years and has served as an administrator in faith community nursing for 10 years. Her dissertation study was focused on parish nursing education, administration, and practice. She has published articles on parish nursing practice, completed a number of research studies on parish nursing practice and outcomes, and provided numerous presentations on faith community nursing. She is active in several professional organizations.

Katora P. Campbell, DrPHc, MSN, RN, CHES
Parish Nurse Manager, Parish Nurse Program, Midlands Partnership for Community Health, Columbia, South Carolina
Dr. Campbell supervises the work of parish nurses serving 19 churches, including the oversight of parish nurse services for low-income senior apartments. In 2001, she received the Excellence in Nursing Award from Sigma Theta Tau at Clemson University for her pioneering work in parish nursing. She is currently completing a doctorate degree in health services policy and management from the University of South Carolina.

Sheila Carroll, MSN, RN, APRN-C, FCN
Director, Rose Garden Center for Hope and Healing, Covington, Kentucky
With a varied nursing career Ms. Carroll changed direction upon graduation as a family nurse practitioner in 1995 from the University of Kentucky. Experience in family practice and emergency medicine led her to another phase of nursing. In October 2009, in cooperation with St. Elizabeth Healthcare in Covington, Kentucky, the Rose Garden Center for Hope and Healing was begun to serve the medically indigent in the Northern Kentucky area. What began as a health ministry continues as the Center grows into a team of an all-volunteer staff in a free clinic led by faith.

Nancy L. Rago Durbin, MS, RN, FCN
Director, Parish Nurse Ministry and Parish Nurse Support Network, Advocate Health Care, Park Ridge, Illinois
With more than 22 years of experience in health ministry, Ms. Durbin has been a leader in developing resources for faith community nursing that include policies, procedures, competencies, program evaluation, and data measurement. She is active in several professional organizations, including Health Ministries Association, and is currently chair of the Faith Community Nurse Recognition Task Force, which works with the American Nurses Credentialing Center and Health Ministries Association to develop a certification process for the specialty practice of faith community nursing.

Marlene Feagan, MA, BSN, RN, FCN
Health Ministries Coordinator, St. Elizabeth Healthcare, Northern Kentucky
For more than 15 years, Ms. Feagan has worked as a health ministries and faith community nursing coordinator. She developed, implemented, and manages a wholistic wellness and prevention model of care for faith

communities and the community at large. She also developed a unique wholistic-based geriatric care management model. She is active in several professional organizations and holds leadership positions for the Health Ministries Association. She has presented and written on health ministries, faith community nursing, spirituality in nursing, and aging issues locally, regionally, and nationally.

Paulette Golden, MS, RN, FCN
Manager, Community Health and Faith Community Nursing Programs, Texas Health Harris Methodist Hospital, Fort Worth, Texas
With more than 30 years nursing experience in a variety of settings of critical care, occupational health, education, and community health, Ms. Golden has worked in the area of faith community nursing for the past nine years. She is active in several professional organizations, including leadership positions in the Texas State Health Ministries Association and the Parish Nurse Faculty through the International Parish Nurse Resources Center.

Beverly Lunsford, PhD, CNS-BC, RN
Associate Research Professor, School of Nursing, The George Washington University, Washington, D.C.
Dr. Lunsford has more than 35 years experience in nursing practice, education, administration, and research. She has taught nursing courses, including research, theory, population health, spirituality and health, and palliative care nursing. Dr. Lunsford has developed new programs for wholistic adolescent and young adult health care and palliative care. She writes grants to fund research and healthcare programs, especially to improve health care for underserved, vulnerable, and disenfranchised populations. She currently directs two grant-funded research projects in geriatric education.

Vickie L. Morley, MSN, RN, FCN
Faith Community Nurse Coordinator, Shenandoah University, Winchester, Virginia
Mrs. Morley has 30 years of nursing experience in a variety of practice settings. Specialty practices include pediatrics, faith community nursing, academia, and continuing education. She has a wealth of experience in faith community nursing as an educator and practitioner. As a national speaker, advocate, and educator, Mrs. Morley is passionate about promoting the specialty practice of faith community nursing.

Katia Reinert, MSN, CRNP, FCN-BC, PHCNS-BC
Family Nurse Practitioner, Smith Ho Internal Medicine; Health Ministries Director, Seventh-Day Adventist Church in North America, Silver Spring, Maryland
Prior to accepting the call to serve in her current role, Ms. Reinert served in the nursing profession at Washington Adventist Hospital for 15 years as a critical care nurse, occupational health nurse practitioner, Faith Community Nursing Coordinator, and Health Ministry Clinical Supervisor for Adventist HealthCare. She fostered medical–religious partnerships and coordinated faith community nursing and lay health ministry training for health professionals and lay ministers. She is currently pursuing doctoral studies in the area of religion and health.

Marilyn Seiler, MS, RN, FCN
Parish Nurse Coordinator, Catholic Parish of St. John the Baptist, Edmond, Oklahoma, and Catholic Parishes of Stillwater, Oklahoma
While serving as the Parish Nurse Coordinator for three Catholic parishes, Ms. Seiler has also been active in providing foundation and ongoing education for faith community nurses in Oklahoma. She has 27 years experience in all types and all positions of home care agencies. In addition, she was a home health consultant with an emphasis in documentation, quality, and general administrative issues. She has authored publications related to home health and faith community nursing.

Roberta Schweitzer, PhD, RN, FCN
Assistant Professor, School of Nursing, College of Health and Human Science, Purdue University, West Lafayette, Indiana; Education Director, Greater Lafayette Parish Nurse Development Center, Lafayette, Indiana
Dr. Schweitzer's 35 years of nursing experience include advanced practice, academic education, and research. For 20 years, she has been involved in the development of faith community nursing practice. Dr. Schweitzer served on the editorial staff for three editions of the International Parish Nurse Resource Center's Foundations of Faith Community Nursing curriculum. Currently, Dr. Schweitzer's faith community nursing practice and education guide her research trajectory as well as her data-based, peer-reviewed publications in nursing journals which focus on spiritual leadership in faith community nursing, spiritual well-being, and health-related quality of life in coping with chronic illness.

Angela Sheehan, MS, RN, FCN
Director, Faith Community/Parish Nurse Program, Seton Health, Troy, New York
As a nurse working for 37 years in many settings, Ms. Sheehan's primary focus in care delivery has become spirituality in nursing. After obtaining a CNS in mental health, she completed coursework for Nurse Practitioner in mental health in 2007. She is dedicated to faith community nursing and believes that mental health and spirituality need to be better integrated, as well as the physical aspects, for a truly holistic healthcare model. Ms. Sheehan believes the art of nursing can be actualized through faith community nursing and works tirelessly to integrate spirituality in all that nurses do.

Norma R. Small, PhD, APRN
Historian, Health Ministries Association, Arnold, Maryland
Dr. Small has more than 50 years experience in nursing practice, education, and administration. She was a founding member of the Health Ministries Association (HMA) and was HMA's consultant for obtaining the American Nurses Association's recognition of parish nursing as a specialty. She was involved in the first publication of *Scope and Standards of Parish Nursing Practice* (HMA, 1998). In 1990, she started the first graduate program in parish health nursing at Georgetown University. Dr. Small currently consults and lectures in the areas of health ministry and faith community nursing.

Sharon Stanton, MS, RN, FCN
Coordinator, Center for Health Ministries, Catholic Healthcare West–Arizona, Chandler, Arizona
Specializing in leadership development, Ms. Stanton has almost 50 years of experience. She has worked in multiple diverse roles integrating public health, migrant health, home health, and academia. Ms. Stanton has worked in the field of faith health ministry for more than 16 years developing best-practice models in the Southeast and Southwest. She currently coordinates and oversees Catholic Healthcare West–Arizona's replicable model for faith health ministry, a collaboration between two major hospitals and 19 faith communities. The model integrates faith community nursing into the total patient care team, provides continuity of care, and increases the potential for data retrieval and research. Ms. Stanton is a cojourner of the Sisters of Saint Francis.

Chris VanDenburgh, MSN, RN, FCN
Coordinator, Faith Community Nursing and Health Ministry, Kettering Health Network, Kettering, Ohio
In addition to faith community nursing, Ms. VanDenburgh's areas of training include clinical pastoral education and critical incident stress management. She has been involved in faith community nursing for many years, both as a full-time, paid faith community nurse and as an educator and program coordinator. Ms. VanDenburgh serves as the Director of Health Ministry for her denominational organization and has been a speaker and presenter on spiritual care, spirituality and healing, and faith community nursing both in the United States and abroad.

Denise Viker, BSN, RN, FCN
Director of Congregational Health Services, Duet, Phoenix, Arizona
Ms. Viker has more than 25 years of experience teaching and managing nurses in a variety of nursing specialties. She has served as a faith community nurse at Desert Cross Lutheran Church in Tempe, Arizona, for more than 10 years. She applies this experience in her role as director by educating and supporting a network of faith community nurses throughout the state of Arizona. She is working collaboratively with students from Arizona State University to develop a faith community nursing database.

Susan Ward, PhD, RN
Nursing Professor, Nebraska Methodist College, Josie Harper Campus, Omaha, Nebraska
Dr. Ward has been an educator for 21 years in undergraduate and graduate nursing programs at Nebraska Methodist College. She has been instrumental at the local, regional, and national levels in moving faith community nursing practice forward. She served as a faith community nurse at Countryside Community Church in Omaha, Nebraska. Her work includes presenting at conferences related to spirituality and health, editing the International Parish Nurse Resource Center (IPNRC) curriculum and foundational documents for global Parish Nurse Resource Centers in conjunction with the IPNRC, and serving on the work group for the 2005 edition of *Faith Community Nursing: Scope and Standards of Practice*. She has presented at professional engagements and taught Nebraska Methodist College's online parish nursing course for more than 10 years.

Appendix A. Faith Community Nursing: Scope and Standards of Practice, Second Edition (2012)

Andrea M. West, PhD, RN, FCN

Director of Curriculum and Research, International Parish Nurse Resource Center, St. Louis, Missouri

Dr. West has more than 25 years experience in nursing education at the diploma, baccalaureate, and graduate levels, including serving as dean of a baccalaureate program. She has served on a variety of nursing and university committees and has been active in the American Nurses Association through the Oklahoma Nurses Association, in the National League for Nursing through the Oklahoma League for Nursing, and in Sigma Theta Tau. Her community activities include membership on a regional hospital board and a three-level care community for the elderly. She coordinated the education program for faith community nursing in Oklahoma.

Paula White, BSN, MSA, RN, FCN

Faith Community Nursing Coordinator, Borgess Health, Kalamazoo, Michigan

With more than 40 years of varied nursing experience across the continuum of care, Ms. White has been active in parish nursing since 1991. Since 2004, she has coordinated Borgess Health's outreach to assist nurses in beginning and sustaining congregational health ministries in nine counties of southwest Michigan. She is a member of the American Nurses Association, Sigma Theta Tau, and the Health Ministries Association. She is an active member of the International Parish Nurse Resource Center faculty, teaching the foundations of faith community nursing, and is a founding member and the treasurer of the West Michigan Partners in Health Ministry.

Diana Williams, MSN, RN, FCN

Director, Community Resources, Our Lady of Bellefonte Hospital, Bon Secours Kentucky Health System, Ashland, Kentucky

Under Ms. Williams's leadership, Our Lady of Bellefonte Hospital was the first organization in its service area to offer health ministry–faith community nursing to local congregations. Since its inception in the fall of 1996, the ministry has developed partnerships with approximately 50 congregations. Ms. Williams is a fellow of the Kentucky Public Health Leadership Institute and the Bon Secours Ministry Leadership Formation Intensive. She is a member of both the Bon Secours and the Kentucky Parish Nurse Networks.

Deborah Ziebarth, MSN, RN, FCN
Assistant Professor of Nursing, Herzing University, Brookfield Campus, Milwaukee, Wisconsin

With more than 30 years of experience in nursing, Ms. Ziebarth has worked extensively in the areas of community health, global health, and academic education. She received national recognition for her management of community-based nursing programs (the American Hospital Association's 2006 Nova Award and the Volunteer Hospital Association's 2008 Best in Class Award). She was recognized in 2010 by Wisconsin Nursing Association with a Face of Nursing Award and recently published the Wisconsin Parish Nurse Minimum Educational Standards, which includes her research. Active on the Wisconsin Parish Nurse Coalition Board, she has held the position of education chair since 2003. She has consulted with the International Parish Nurse Resource Center on various projects. Recently, Ms. Ziebarth joined Herzing University as a member of the nursing faculty.

ANA Staff

Carol Bickford, PhD, RN-BC, CPHIMS – Content editor
Yvonne Daley Humes, MSA – Project coordinator
Maureen E. Cones, Esq. – Legal counsel
Eric Wurzbacher –Project editor
Melaney Johnson –Printing and manufacturing coordinator

About the American Nurses Association

The American Nurses Association (ANA) is the only full-service professional organization representing the interests of the nation's 3.1 million registered nurses through its constituent/state nurses associations and its organizational affiliates. The ANA advances the nursing profession by fostering high standards of nursing practice, promoting the rights of nurses in the workplace, projecting a positive and realistic view of nursing, and lobbying the Congress and regulatory agencies on healthcare issues affecting nurses and the public. More at www.NursingWorld.org.

Appendix A. Faith Community Nursing: Scope and Standards of Practice, Second Edition (2012)

About Health Ministries Association, Inc.

Health Ministries Association, Inc. (HMA), a nonprofit membership organization, is a support network for people of faith who promote whole-person health through faith groups in the communities they serve. HMA is the recognized professional membership organization for the nursing specialty of faith community nursing and promotes education, research utilization, and evidence-based practice. By providing information, guidelines, and resources, HMA assists and encourages individuals, families, and communities as they develop whole-person health programs, utilize community resources, and educate others on the interdependent health of body, mind, and spirit. More at www.hmassoc.org/.

About Nursesbooks.org, The Publishing Program of ANA

Nursesbooks.org publishes books on ANA core issues and programs, including ethics, leadership, quality, specialty practice, advanced practice, and the profession's enduring legacy. Best known for the foundational documents of the profession on ethics, scope and standards of practice, and social policy, Nursesbooks.org is the publisher for the professional, career-oriented nurse, reaching and serving nurse educators, administrators, managers, and researchers, as well as staff nurses in the course of their professional development. More at www.Nursesbooks.org/.

Appendix A. Faith Community Nursing: Scope and Standards of Practice, Second Edition (2012)

Introduction

The American Nurses Association (ANA) published the first *Scope and Standards of Parish Nursing Practice* in 1998. As the practice of parish nursing evolved, the title of the specialty practice was changed to *faith community nursing* with the publication of *Faith Community Nursing: Scope and Standards of Practice* in 2005. Since then, there have been dramatic changes in health care as well as the nursing profession. *Faith Community Nursing: Scope and Standards of Practice, Second Edition,* describes the specialty practice of faith community nursing for the nursing profession, faith community nurses, other healthcare providers, spiritual leaders, employers, insurers, healthcare consumers, families, and members of faith communities. The unique scope of knowledge and the standards of practice and professional performance for a faith community nurse (FCN) are discussed.

Function of the Scope of Practice Statement of Faith Community Nursing

The scope of practice statement describes the *who, what, where, when, why,* and *how* of the practice of faith community nursing. The answers to these questions provide a complete picture of the practice, its boundaries, and its membership. *Nursing: Scope and Standards of Practice, Second Edition* (ANA, 2010a) applies to all professional registered nurses engaged in practice, regardless of specialty, practice setting, or educational preparation. With *Code of Ethics for Nurses with Interpretive Statements* (ANA, 2001) and *Nursing's Social Policy Statement: The Essence of the Profession* (ANA, 2010b), it forms the foundation of practice for all registered nurses. The scope of faith community nursing practice is specific to this specialty but builds on the scope of practice expected of all registered nurses.

Function of the Standards of Faith Community Nursing Practice

Standards are "authoritative statements defined and promoted by the profession by which the quality of practice, service, or education can be evaluated" (ANA, 2010a, p. 67). Standards reflect the values and priorities of the profession and provide direction for professional nursing practice and a framework for evaluation of this practice. The standards of faith community nursing practice are specific to this specialty but build on the standards of professional nursing practice applicable to all registered nurses.

Development of *Faith Community Nursing: Scope and Standards of Practice, Second Edition*

Health Ministries Association (HMA), the professional membership organization for nurses in this specialty, and ANA collaborated in the development and publication of *Faith Community Nursing: Scope and Standards of Practice* in 2005. With the publication of *Nursing: Scope and Standards of Practice, Second Edition* (ANA, 2010a), all specialty scope and standards of practice are now being revised. For continuity and consistency, that publication was used as the template when developing this new edition.

Following the 2005 revision, the HMA board requested volunteers to serve on a working group to review and revise the scope and standards for faith community nursing. Twenty-one practicing nurses representing different areas of the country and various roles in this specialty practice contributed to this revision. A draft copy of the document was posted on the HMA web site for public review. Responses were received and carefully considered in creating the final document. As a result, this document provides a national perspective on the current practice of this specialty of faith community nursing.

Summary

The scope and standards of practice for faith community nursing reflect the commitment of the Health Ministries Association to work with the American Nurses Association to promote an understanding of faith community nursing as a specialized practice in the interprofessional practice arena of diverse faith communities. HMA is the national professional organization representing faith community nurses and others working in the expanding faith community arena.

As the diversity of participating faith communities expands in rural areas, towns, and cities, the difficulty in finding all-inclusive terminology to describe the beliefs and practices that have evolved from the variety of traditions becomes more apparent. Terms used in this document indicate an effort to include many faith traditions and not to promote any one particular faith tradition.

Faith Community Nursing: Scope and Standards of Practice, Second Edition, reflects current faith community nursing practice from a national perspective, the professional and ethical standards of the nursing profession, and the legal scope and standards of professional nursing practice. They are dynamic and subject to testing and change.

Scope of Faith Community Nursing Practice

Definition and Overview of Faith Community Nursing

Faith community nursing is a specialized practice of professional nursing that focuses on the intentional care of the spirit as well as on the promotion of wholistic health and prevention or minimization of illness within the context of a faith community.

The term *faith community nurse* (FCN) is used to represent a registered nurse specializing in faith community nursing. The FCN is knowledgeable in two primary areas—professional nursing and spiritual care. The faith community nurse provides spiritual care in the faith community as well as in the broader community. The goals of an FCN are the protection, promotion, and optimization of health and abilities; the prevention of illness and injury; and the alleviation of suffering in the context of the values, beliefs, and practices of a faith community, such as a church, congregation, parish, synagogue, temple, mosque, or faith-based community agency.

Healthcare consumer is the term used by the American Nurses Association to define a person, client, family, group, community, or population that is the focus of attention and to which the registered nurse is providing services as sanctioned by the state regulatory bodies. In narratives within the specialty of faith community nursing, other terms such as *parishioner, congregant,* or *faith community member* may also be included as descriptive terms. The term *healthcare consumer* may refer to the faith community as a whole, or to groups, families, and individuals in the faith community. People from the broader community may also seek the services of the FCN.

The FCN uses the nursing process to address the spiritual, physical, mental, and social health of the healthcare consumer. With an intentional focus on spiritual health, the FCN primarily uses the interventions of education, counseling, prayer, presence, active listening, advocacy, referral, and a wide variety of resources available to the faith community. The faith community nurse may also train and supervise volunteers from the faith community. As an actively licensed registered nurse, the FCN provides nursing care based on standards and professional experience, legal expectations, and education. The FCN focuses on the needs of the healthcare consumer population and the position as defined by the faith community. The FCN collaborates with other specialties, such as primary care, community health, hospice, rehabilitation, home health, acute care, critical care, integrative health, and long-term care in other aspects of care for the faith community and its members.

This document—in conjunction with *Nursing's Social Policy Statement: The Essence of the Profession* (ANA, 2010b), *Nursing: Scope and Standards of Practice, Second Edition* (ANA, 2010a), and *Code of Ethics for Nurses with Interpretive Statements* (ANA, 2001)—delineates the professional responsibilities of an FCN. FCNs are also bound by the laws, statutes, and regulations related to nursing practice for their state, commonwealth, or territory.

Evolution of Faith Community Nursing

Nursing has its historical foundation deeply rooted in faith and health, as well as in the ancient and recent traditions of many religions. Faith traditions established rules for public health, including care of persons with infectious diseases. These communities also included visiting the sick and caring for infants and the elderly as religious duty. This sense of duty to care for a community's members expanded to include "care for the stranger" and was the basis for early *diakonas*—houses for strangers—which became the first charity hospitals. In the 12th, 13th, and 14th centuries, a new cadre of men serving in nursing orders emerged and provided care to men and women wounded in wars and to lepers. Religious orders also provided care for persons with mental illnesses. During the 16th century, more than 100 female religious orders were founded specifically to do nursing.

The faith and health link evolved over time and has been influenced by cultural, political, social, and economic events. Religious groups founded hospitals to provide care to vulnerable populations, such as the poor, immigrant, and homeless. In the late 1800s churches began to reclaim their role in healing. Diaconal ministries that developed in Europe migrated to the United States, and immigrant churches imported the work of deaconesses and other religious orders to provide health care to those in their communities. These religious affiliations were instrumental in developing schools of nursing during the 20th century.

Florence Nightingale, trained through the Deaconess Institution in Kaiserswerth, Germany, felt called to the service of the sick. In addition to her nursing education, she was a theological scholar and writer. Her religious philosophy and belief in a higher power was the foundation for her work to promote nursing as a trained profession, establish a public healthcare system that included health promotion and preventive medicine, and advocate for health issues as a social activist. The rich history of nursing's evolution is exquisitely collected in Patricia Donahue's (1996) *Nursing, The Finest Art: An Illustrated History*.

In the late 1950s, Halbert Dunn, a physician, developed a public health concept that he called high-level wellness. His writings were a catalyst for wellness centers that began in the 1970s. A growing public interest in complementary and alternative medicine influenced Western conventional medical care to incorporate aspects of these models into integrated care. This growing interest and focus on health promotion and wellness influenced the development of faith community nursing.

In 1979, Rev. Dr. Granger Westberg created wholistic health centers in Christian congregations, staffed by a treatment/healing team, comprising a doctor, a nurse, a social worker, and a pastoral counselor. The nurses in these centers were referred to as "parish nurses." Since then various other faith communities have established programs of health and healing led by a registered nurse. The word "parish" in *parish nurse* is not appropriate in all faith traditions, so faith communities have created different titles for this specialized nursing role. To have one name inclusive of all faith traditions and to accurately label the location and focus of practice, the specialty practice described in this document is *faith community nursing*. In a given setting, the faith community nurse may be referred to as a *parish nurse, congregational nurse, health ministry nurse, crescent nurse*, or *health and wellness nurse*.

Westberg used the term *wholistic health* to define a whole or completely integrated approach to health and health care that integrates the physical and spiritual aspects of the whole person. The principles of wholistic health arose from the understanding that human beings strive for wholeness in their relationship to their God or higher power, themselves, their families, the society, and the environment in which they live. Based on its historic meaning, *wholistic* is the preferred spelling when referring to the health care provided by faith community nurses.

Nurse-led programs within and beyond Judeo-Christian faith communities continue to grow and evolve. The common expectation across faith traditions is that the professional registered nurse functioning as an FCN possesses a depth of understanding of the faith community's traditions, as well as competence as a registered nurse, using the nursing process so that the nursing care integrates care of the spirit with care of the body and mind.

Assumptions of Faith Community Nursing

These five assumptions underlie faith community nursing:

- Health and illness are human experiences.

- Health is the integration of the spiritual, physical, psychological, and social aspects of the healthcare consumer to create a sense of harmony with self, others, the environment, and a higher power.

- Health may be experienced in the presence of disease or injury.

- The presence of illness does not preclude health nor does optimal health preclude illness.

- Healing is the process of integrating the body, mind, and spirit to create wholeness, health, and a sense of well-being, even when the healthcare consumer's illness is not cured.

Focusing on Spiritual Care in Nursing

Nurses have long observed that when illness or brokenness occurs, healthcare consumers—whether individually or with their family or friends—may turn to their source of spiritual strength for reassurance, support, and healing. *Nursing: Scope and Standards of Practice, Second Edition* (ANA, 2010a) reaffirms that spiritual care is a part of all nursing practice. The primary focus of the FCN is the intentional care of the spirit, differentiating this specialty practice from the general practice of a registered nurse. Within this specialized knowledge base, each FCN will demonstrate competence on a continuum of expertise.

A variety of tools for spiritual assessment have been developed and tested for reliability and validity. These tools, varying from simple screening to in-depth assessments, are increasingly used in nursing practice. Because, in general, the use of spiritual assessment tools has not been taught to providers from other disciplines, the FCN may provide leadership to the staff in the selection and application of assessment tools.

After analyzing the assessment data, the FCN selects the diagnoses to describe actual or potential needs of the healthcare consumer, including spiritual needs. These diagnoses then provide the basis for interventions to achieve the outcomes for which the nurse is accountable.

Treatment may or may not cure an affliction. However, it is still possible through care of the spirit for a person to be healed even if a cure—physical restoration—does not occur. A person may be dying from cancer, but if a broken relationship between family members has been reconciled or the person is at peace with the circumstances, this may be considered healing.

Assault, betrayal, accident, or death of a member of the community can affect an entire faith community. Members of all ages may manifest anger, grief, depression, anxiety, fear, and spiritual or physical pain in varying degrees. An FCN's response to such an event is complex. Beyond identifying and meeting the needs of individuals and families, the FCN treats the whole-faith community as a healthcare consumer. Assessment focuses on identifying the educational and supportive needs of the whole-faith community. Interventions occur at three different levels: community, family or group, and individual.

The FCN will address a variety of issues that threaten the wholistic health of persons in the faith community:

- Individuals or families may lack food, shelter, transportation, income, or health care.

- Victims of violence, abuse, or exploitation in a variety of settings, including domestic settings, may seek solace or sanctuary.

- Adult children of aging parents may seek guidance in talking with or determining the appropriate living situation for a parent, and ongoing assistance from the faith community.

- Victims of natural disasters and other life-altering emergencies may require various forms of assistance.

To respond to these and other situations wholistically, an FCN draws on professional skills that integrate spiritual care and nursing care, as well as the resources of individuals and groups both within and beyond the faith community, to provide a wholistic response. Some healthcare consumers will require support of basic needs so that they have the time and space to reflect on spiritual issues; for others, spiritual care will be the direct response. The form of spiritual care will depend on the beliefs and practices of the faith community; the desire of the faith community, the group, or the individual; the skills of the FCN; and the collaboration of other staff members and volunteers.

Health Advocacy and Faith Community Nursing

One of the key aspects of faith community nursing is health advocacy. As stated in *Code of Ethics for Nurses with Interpretive Statements* (ANA, 2001, p. 16), the faith community nurse "promotes, advocates for, and strives to protect the health, safety, and rights of the patient." In the settings for faith community nursing, this often includes advocating for appropriate levels of care for vulnerable populations and those with limited access to healthcare resources. Such advocacy may include initiating referrals for clinical treatment, obtaining home care resources, or assisting with extended care arrangements. Faith community nurses may promote advocacy for healthcare consumers with low health literacy skills by accompanying them to provider appointments and providing health education in more readily understood terminology. Faith community nurses participate in promoting community awareness of significant health problems and building community coalitions of faith-based and service organizations to stimulate supportive public policy and interprofessional beneficial actions for improving health.

Educational Preparation for Faith Community Nursing

The faith community nurse bridges two domains and thus must be prepared in and responsible for both nursing and spiritual care. This document provides a comprehensive picture of this specialty practice as such and as part of the nursing profession. Each faith tradition may provide additional stipulations and requirements. There are designations in the specialty that indicate the level of education achieved.

Faith community nurses may also have graduate- and doctoral-level preparation in clinical nursing specialties, theology, clinical spiritual care, complementary care, palliative care, and wholistic health.

Appropriate and effective practice as an FCN requires the ability to integrate current nursing, behavioral, environmental, and spiritual knowledge with the unique spiritual beliefs and religious practices of the faith community into a program of wholistic nursing care. Such integrative practice is required regardless of the academic education of the nurse. With education, mentoring, and a collaborative practice site, an FCN may progress in levels of expertise in this specialty practice.

Faith Community Nurse

The preferred minimum preparation for a registered nurse or advanced practice registered nurse entering the specialty of faith community nursing includes:

- A baccalaureate or higher degree in nursing with academic preparation in community- or population-focused nursing

- Experience as a registered nurse using the nursing process

- Knowledge of the healthcare assets and resources of the community

- Specialized knowledge of the spiritual beliefs and practices of the faith community

- Specialized knowledge and skills to enable implementation of *Faith Community Nursing: Scope and Standards of Practice, Second Edition*

Currently, the education of all nursing students preparing for the national examination for RN licensure includes basic content on spiritual care. In addition, an increasing number of undergraduate students during their community health courses participate in clinical experiences with faith community nurses. However, because of the intentional focus on spiritual care by the faith community nurse, this educational exposure is not adequate preparation for assuming the specialty role of an FCN.

A registered nurse may prepare for the specialty of faith community nursing in several ways. Preparation may occur through accredited continuing education programs, a baccalaureate program, or graduate nursing courses.

A national Health Ministries Association (HMA) task force initiated work with the American Nurses Credentialing Center (ANCC) to begin defining criteria and a process for formal recognition of faith community nursing. Although this work is not yet completed, one of its outcomes was to establish 34 contact hours of continuing education content specific to faith community nursing as the minimum course length for the preparation for this nursing specialty.

Some educational institutions that specialize in religious education also offer relevant courses or programs of study. Collaboration between disciplines has also led to offering dual master's degrees in nursing and either theology or health ministry. Mentoring during an orientation period can also enhance faith community nursing practice. Faith communities understand, support, and often fund continuing education and spiritual development for FCNs to enhance their ability to provide spiritual care, knowing that this directly benefits a community's own programs.

Graduate-prepared or theologically prepared nurses may have certifications associated with their educational major. Currently, the motivation for a faith community nurse to pursue certification is self-directed and encouraged as part of demonstrating competence in the specialty. A specialty certification process for faith community nursing is not now available, but has been initiated as part of a pilot project. In December 2007, HMA began working with ANCC to develop a portfolio assessment process for the recognition of faith community nurses. In 2009, the portfolio assessment process was placed on hold for further study. HMA is committed to resuming work with ANCC with the intent that the portfolio process would be available for all faith community nurses interested in formal recognition by ANCC.

Advanced Practice Registered Nurse

By definition, an *advanced practice registered nurse* (APRN) is a nurse who has completed an accredited graduate-level education program preparing her or him for the role of certified nurse practitioner (CNP), certified registered nurse anesthetist (CRNA), certified nurse midwife (CNM), or clinical nurse specialist (CNS); has passed a national certification examination that measures the APRN role and population-focused competencies; maintains continued competence as evidenced by recertification; and is licensed to practice as an APRN.

An emerging role in healthcare delivery models is that of an APRN and other graduate-level prepared nurses who have acquired the additional specialized education for practice as a faith community nurse. These nurses integrate theoretical and evidence-based knowledge from graduate nursing education with the specialized education of an FCN regarding the structure, spiritual beliefs, and practices of the faith group. Examples that illustrate this role include a CNP, a wound-ostomy nurse CNS, an oncology CNS, a palliative care CNS, and a mental health CNS practicing in a faith-based community clinic.

Besides providing nursing care, these APRNs influence nursing care outcomes by serving as an advocate, consultant, or researcher in the specialty area, by providing expert consultation for spiritual leaders and other healthcare providers, and by identifying and facilitating improvements in wholistic health care.

APRN is a regulatory title and includes the four roles (CNP, CRNA, CNM, and CNS). The core competencies for education and the scope of practice are defined by the professional associations. State law and regulation further define criteria for licensure for the designated scopes of practice.

Additional Designations

National leaders of faith groups that recognize the importance of integrating this specialty nursing practice into faith communities have developed mechanisms for mentoring and providing informal and formal education in the concepts of spiritual beliefs, practices, and rituals. When such mechanisms are available within the faith group, the FCN may work with the leadership of the faith community to meet the educational and practice requirements to earn formal designation as a spiritual leader in the particular faith group.

Faith groups have different ways of designating or titling individuals who have attained an advanced level of preparation and often undergone examination to determine fitness for providing spiritual care. FCNs who achieve the requirements defined by the faith group in which they are practicing may then be given a title by the faith community indicating their achievement, such as *deacon, minister of health,* or *pastoral associate.* Titles such as these have a specialized meaning within the faith community served.

Competence and Competency in Faith Community Nursing

The American Nurses Association identifies that in the practice of nursing, "competence is definable, measurable and can be evaluated. Competence is situational, dynamic, and is both an outcome and an ongoing process. Competency is an expected level of performance that integrates knowledge, skills, abilities, and judgment in formal, informal, and reflective learning experiences. Knowledge encompasses thinking, understanding of science and humanities, professional standards of practice, and insights gained from practical experiences, personal capabilities, and leadership performance. Context determines what competencies are necessary" (ANA, 2010a, p. 12). "Formal learning most often occurs in structured, academic, and professional development environments, while informal learning can be described as experiential insights gained in work, community, home, and other settings. Reflective learning represents the recurrent thoughtful personal self-assessment, analysis, and synthesis of strengths and opportunities for improvement" (ANA, 2010a, p. 13).

Faith community nurses integrate cognitive, psychomotor, communication, interpersonal, and diagnostic skills. Their ability to act effectively involves active listening, integrity, knowledge of one's strengths and weaknesses, positive self-regard, emotional intelligence, spiritual formation, and openness to feedback. Faith community nurses must continually reassess their competencies and identify needs for additional knowledge, skills, personal growth, and integrative learning experiences.

Competence in faith community nursing practice must be evaluated by the individual nurse, peers, mentors, and faith community leaders. No single evaluation method or tool can guarantee competence. The Health Ministries Association, in its work with ANCC, has developed sources of evidence such as evidence-based case studies, spiritual journey and leadership templates, peer evaluations, faith community member narratives, and evidence of faith community nursing educational preparation and continuing education.

Settings for Practice in Faith Community Nursing

An FCN serves as a member of the interprofessional staff of a faith community, providing care to the faith community as a whole, as well as to member groups and individuals. The FCN is often the only healthcare provider responsible for practice in this nontraditional healthcare setting, although others from the faith community assist the FCN. In many circumstances, the FCN works in partnership with community agencies and healthcare systems.

Most encounters between healthcare consumers and FCNs are initiated within the faith community settings, programs, or healthcare consumers' homes. Participants in the various activities of the faith community may seek the services of the FCN. These activities include worship, education, healing prayer, special interest or support groups, programs for spiritual growth or renewal, and support services, such as shelters and soup kitchens.

A community of faith may be composed of people of all ages. The FCN provides wholistic nursing care to pediatric, adolescent, adult, and geriatric members of the faith community. The members may also represent a diverse range of physical, emotional, and cognitive development. When an individual, family, group, or the faith community as a whole experiences or desires a change in their level of physical, mental, social, environmental, or spiritual well-being, or when maintaining their current level of well-being requires nursing action, an FCN collaborates with them to develop a plan of care that incorporates communal and individual spiritual beliefs and practices.

The FCN monitors environmental, hygiene, and safety issues of faith community facilities and chooses appropriate responses in collaboration with the leadership of the faith community. Examples include hygiene and safety protocols for day care centers and nurseries; infection control during worship, health fairs, or blood drives; and protocols for response to medical emergencies. The FCN also manages physical and mental health issues, including the high levels of stress of spiritual leaders, other staff members, or faith community volunteers, with interventions that encompass spiritual support, health promotion, illness prevention, and disease management.

The needs and desires of individual members of the faith community may require that the FCN visit members in a hospital or hospice, private home, or residential facility, or accompany healthcare consumers as they use health services within the community. During these encounters the FCN may also intervene with spiritual care and provide a supportive, healing presence for both the healthcare consumer and loved ones.

The size, concerns, assets, and expectations of the faith community will guide the development of the expected role of an FCN. As a staff member, the FCN is most often supported and guided by a committee of faith community leaders and assisted by lay volunteers. With education and supervision provided by the FCN, these volunteers may assume tasks that family members would do for each other if they were available. This type of supportive team, led by the FCN, can increase safety and comfort during hospital discharge transitions and provide healthcare consumers with comprehensive support once home, helping them to recuperate more easily or to achieve peace before death.

Continued Commitment to the Profession

Because the specialty practice of faith community nursing is relatively new, each FCN needs to educate other healthcare providers and the general public about the benefits of this type of nursing care. An FCN may participate with faith community colleagues to develop collaborative efforts throughout the community by joining, for instance, a faith community nurses' group or a clergy association.

The FCN commits to lifelong learning in nursing, spiritual growth, and the beliefs and practices of the faith community. There are numerous opportunities for personal and professional growth both in and beyond the community. Major denominations support both programs and professional development. The professional organization for faith community nurses, Health Ministries Association, provides opportunities for networking and ongoing education in the practice specialty as well as with other disciplines. A variety of educational institutions and resource centers is also available around the country or online.

While the FCN may be the only healthcare provider in the faith community, the best practice cannot be provided in isolation. Personal and professional support, education opportunities, and resources are available. Accessing these will improve both the care provided to the faith community and the progress of the specialty.

Research and Faith Community Nursing

Research conducted at the National Institutes of Health and academic institutions has established a relationship between spiritual practices and health, thereby expanding the knowledge base for the specialty of faith community nursing. Findings from a variety of nonnursing disciplines provide understanding of the strong connection between spiritual well-being, participation in religious practices, and wholistic health. Involvement in a faith community provides health benefits through social support, a social identity, and a sense of power beyond one's self. Religious and spiritual practices, such as meditation, prayer, and touch, are reported to lengthen life, improve the quality of life, and improve health outcomes by enhancing psychological, physical, and spiritual well-being. Research reports may be found in the nursing literature and publications of other health professionals, as well as the professional literature focused on health ministry, chaplaincy, theology, spirituality, and spiritual care.

Research by faith community nurses to evaluate the benefits of this specialty practice is emerging. Recent studies include investigations of the measurement of clinical outcomes and the cost–benefits of faith community nursing interventions, and descriptive studies of FCN models of practice. Funding would enhance efforts to establish programs of collaborative research between practicing faith community nurses and nurse researchers that could validate and promote the wholistic health benefits of this nursing specialty in the interprofessional environment. Confirmation of positive outcomes is a major influence in funding further research and positions for faith community nurses.

Professional Trends and Issues in Faith Community Nursing

Since 1998, when faith community nursing was formally recognized by the American Nurses Association as a specialty nursing practice, there has been tremendous growth in both professional knowledge and the number of faith communities seeking such services. With this growth several issues have become more apparent.

Titling FCNs so that the title is understood across various faith traditions. This issue has been addressed with the adoption of an all-encompassing title for this specialty, *faith community nursing*. Sensitivity to the desires of individual faith communities to maintain their own internal title has also been considered. Just as each community calls their spiritual leaders by their own titles, such as rabbi, pastor, minister, or teacher, they may also call the FCN by the title they choose. However, selection of an internal title different from faith community nurse does not relieve that registered nurse from fulfilling the expectations set forth in this document.

Identifying the preparation needed for this specialty practice. This discussion is ongoing. When educational resources for this specialty were limited, nurses had minimal opportunities. With the clarification of minimum standards and an increasing awareness by nurse educators and practicing nurses of the requirements for this specialty practice, both educational expectations and opportunities have increased at all levels of nursing education. The Robert Wood Johnson Foundation and the Institute of Medicine publication, *The Future of Nursing: Leading Change, Advancing Health*, emphasizes an "action-oriented blueprint for the future of nursing" and includes recommendations for nursing educational preparation and training (2010).

Engaging other practice disciplines and faith communities in accepting this specialty nursing practice. As the number and professional activities of faith community nurses increase, so too does the recognition of these specialists by other disciplines. Faith community nurses are vital partners in advancing the nation's health initiatives, such as the Healthy People 2020 framework, to increase the quality and years of healthy life and eliminate health disparities. As members of faith communities experience the benefit of care from an FCN and share their experiences with others, the demand for these services will increase.

Developing transitional care. The recent introduction of transitional care in healthcare delivery models reflects an aspect of care that faith community nurses have been providing for members of their faith communities. Models between faith community nurses and healthcare providers are now developing in several locations as examples of collaborative community care.

Creating paid positions so that more professional nurses may choose to enter the specialty. Financial compensation for providing faith community nursing services is a complex subject familiar to those who know the history of compensation in professional nursing. In this case, the issue is complicated by three major factors:

- Lack of financial resources in many faith communities for an expansion of services

- A faith community's tradition of donating time and expertise to care for its members

- Limited objective data that demonstrate the positive health effects and benefits of faith community nursing so that external funding will be more available

As with any complex issue, addressing this situation is a multifaceted process. Some faith community nurses choose to provide care part-time or full-time, at low financial compensation if any, as part of their gift to the faith community. Others provide care so that they may demonstrate the value of this specialty practice and collect data to support the hiring of a faith community nurse for that community of faith. Some nurses, taking a broader perspective, work within faith community organizations to increase recognition of this specialty nursing practice as a form of spiritual leadership worthy of financial support. Still others encourage healthcare organizations and facilities to provide financial support to FCNs in faith communities. Given the varied dynamics of individual communities of faith, there is no one solution.

This document delineates the professional expectations associated with this specialty nursing practice. When it is considered in conjunction with *Nursing's Social Policy Statement: The Essence of the Profession* (ANA, 2010b), *Nursing: Scope and Standards of Practice, Second Edition* (ANA, 2010a), and *Code of Ethics for Nurses with Interpretive Statements* (ANA, 2001), the professional nurse receives clear guidance in the requirements for preparation and practice that best serve the public's health and the nursing profession.

Standards of Faith Community Nursing Practice

The term *faith community nurse* (FCN) is used to represent a registered nurse specializing in faith community nursing.

Standards of Practice for Faith Community Nursing

Standard 1. Assessment

The faith community nurse collects comprehensive data pertinent to the healthcare consumer's wholistic health or the situation.

COMPETENCIES
The faith community nurse:

- Collects wholistic data including but not limited to physical, functional, psychosocial, emotional, cognitive, sexual, cultural, age-related, environmental, economic, and spiritual or transpersonal assessments in a systematic and ongoing process, while honoring the uniqueness of the person and placing a particular emphasis on spiritual beliefs and practices.

- Elicits the healthcare consumer's values, preferences, expressed needs, and knowledge of the healthcare situation.

- Involves the healthcare consumer, family, group, spiritual leader, other healthcare providers, and others, as appropriate, in wholistic data collection.

- Identifies barriers (e.g., psychosocial, literacy, financial, cultural) to effective communication and makes appropriate adaptations.

- Recognizes the impact of personal attitudes, values, and beliefs.

- Assesses family dynamics and impact on healthcare consumer health and wellness.

- Prioritizes data collection activities based on the healthcare consumer's immediate condition, or the anticipated needs of the healthcare consumer or situation.

- Uses appropriate evidence-based assessment techniques and instruments in collecting pertinent data as a basis for wholistic care.

- Synthesizes available data, information, and knowledge relevant to the situation to identify patterns and variances in individuals, families, groups, or the faith community as a whole.

- Applies ethical, legal, and privacy guidelines and policies to the collection, maintenance, uses, and dissemination of data and information.

- Recognizes healthcare consumers as the authority on their own health by honoring their care preferences.

- Documents relevant data in a retrievable format that is both confidential and secure.

ADDITIONAL COMPETENCIES FOR THE GRADUATE-LEVEL PREPARED FAITH COMMUNITY NURSE AND THE ADVANCED PRACTICE REGISTERED NURSE

The graduate-level prepared faith community nurse or advanced practice registered nurse:

- Initiates and interprets results from diagnostic tests relevant to the wholistic assessment of the healthcare consumer's current status.

- Assesses the effect of interactions among individuals, family, community, and social systems on the healthcare consumer's whole (physical, mental, emotional, and spiritual) health and illness.

- Uses evidence-based analytical models and problem-solving tools.

Standard 2. Diagnosis

The faith community nurse analyzes the assessment data to determine the diagnoses or issues.

COMPETENCIES

The faith community nurse:

- Derives the diagnoses or issues from wholistic assessment data.

- Validates the diagnoses or issues with the healthcare consumer, family, spiritual leader, and other healthcare providers, when possible and appropriate.

- Identifies actual, perceived, or potential threats and barriers to wholistic health and spiritual well-being.

- Uses standardized classification systems and clinical decision support tools, when available, in identifying diagnoses.

- Documents diagnoses in a manner that facilitates the determination of the expected outcomes and plan.

- Identifies strengths that enhance health and spiritual well-being.

ADDITIONAL COMPETENCIES FOR THE GRADUATE-LEVEL PREPARED FAITH COMMUNITY NURSE AND THE ADVANCED PRACTICE REGISTERED NURSE

The graduate-level prepared faith community nurse or advanced practice registered nurse:

- Systematically compares and contrasts clinical findings with normal and abnormal variations and developmental events in formulating a differential diagnosis.

- Utilizes complex data and information obtained during interview, wholistic assessment, examination, and diagnostic procedures in identifying diagnoses.

- Assists registered nurses in developing and maintaining competency in the diagnostic process.

Standard 3. Outcomes Identification

The faith community nurse identifies expected outcomes for a plan individualized to the healthcare consumer or the situation.

COMPETENCIES

The faith community nurse:

- Involves the healthcare consumer, family, spiritual leaders, and healthcare providers in formulating expected outcomes when possible and as appropriate.

- Derives culturally and spiritually appropriate expected outcomes from the identified diagnoses.

- Considers spiritual beliefs and practices, associated benefits, costs, risks, current scientific evidence, and clinical expertise when formulating expected outcomes.

- Defines expected outcomes in terms of the healthcare consumer and the healthcare consumer's values, spiritual and faith beliefs and practices, ethical considerations, family perspectives, cultural practices, environment, or situation with considerations such as associated benefits, risks, costs, and current scientific evidence.

- Includes a realistic time estimate for attaining expected outcomes.

- Uses collaborative discussions to develop expected outcomes that provide direction for continuity of care.

- Modifies expected outcomes based on changes in the status or desires of the healthcare consumer or on evaluation of the situation.

- Documents expected outcomes as measurable goals.

- Develops expected outcomes that facilitate attaining, maintaining, or regaining health, healing, and hope.

ADDITIONAL COMPETENCIES FOR THE GRADUATE-LEVEL PREPARED FAITH COMMUNITY NURSE AND THE ADVANCED PRACTICE REGISTERED NURSE

The graduate-level prepared faith community nurse or advanced practice registered nurse:

- Identifies expected outcomes that incorporate scientific evidence and are achievable through implementation of evidence-based practices.

- Identifies expected outcomes that incorporate cost and clinical effectiveness, healthcare consumer spiritual beliefs and satisfaction with care and quality of life, and consistency and continuity among providers.

- Differentiates outcomes that require care process interventions from those that require system-level interventions.

- Supports the use of clinical and spiritual guidelines linked to positive healthcare consumer outcomes of wholistic health and healing.

Standard 4. Planning

The faith community nurse develops a plan that prescribes strategies and alternatives to attain expected outcomes.

COMPETENCIES

The faith community nurse:

- Develops an individualized plan in partnership with the person, family, and others that considers the person's characteristics or situation, including but not limited to values, spiritual beliefs and practices, health practices, preferences, choices, developmental level, coping style, culture, religious rites, environment, and available technology.

- Establishes the plan priorities with the healthcare consumer, family, and others, as appropriate.

- Includes strategies in the plan that address each of the identified diagnoses, issues, and strengths, which may include strategies for promotion and restoration of health; spiritual enhancement; prevention of illness, injury, and disease; alleviation of suffering; and provision of supportive care for those who are dying.

- Includes strategies for health and wholeness across the life span.

- Provides for continuity within the plan.

- Incorporates an implementation pathway or timeline within the plan.

- Considers the economic impact of the plan on the healthcare consumer, family, caregivers, or other affected parties and how the faith community resources and local community resources might be of assistance.

- Integrates current scientific evidence, healthcare and wholistic health trends, and research affecting care in planning.

- Uses the plan to provide direction to other lay and professional members of the healthcare and ministry teams.

- Explores practice settings and safe space and time for the nurse and the healthcare consumer to explore suggested, potential, and alternative options.

- Defines the plan to reflect current statutes, rules, regulations, and standards.

- Modifies the plan according to the ongoing assessment of the healthcare consumer's response and other outcome indicators.

- Documents the plan in a manner that uses standardized language or recognized terminology and is understood by all participants.

- Includes strategies for wholistic health, with a focus on spirituality and growth across the life span.

ADDITIONAL COMPETENCIES FOR THE GRADUATE-LEVEL PREPARED FAITH COMMUNITY NURSE AND THE ADVANCED PRACTICE REGISTERED NURSE

The graduate-level prepared faith community nurse or advanced practice registered nurse:

- Incorporates assessment strategies, diagnostic strategies, and therapeutic interventions that reflect current evidence, including data, research, literature, and expert nursing knowledge to enhance wholistic health.

- Selects or designs nursing strategies to meet the multifaceted wholistic health needs of complex healthcare consumers.

- Includes the synthesis of healthcare consumers' values and spiritual beliefs regarding nursing and medical therapies in the plan.

- Participates in the design and development of interprofessional processes to address the situation or issue.

- Contributes to the development and continuous improvement of organizational systems that support the planning process.

- Supports the integration of clinical, human, and financial resources to enhance and complete the decision-making process.

Standard 5. Implementation

The faith community nurse implements the identified plan.

COMPETENCIES

The faith community nurse:

- Partners with the person, family, significant others, and caregiver to implement the plan in a safe, realistic, and timely manner.

- Demonstrates caring behaviors toward healthcare consumers, significant others, and groups of people receiving care.

- Utilizes technology to measure, record, and retrieve healthcare consumer data, implement the nursing process, and enhance nursing practice.

- Utilizes evidence-based interventions and treatments specific to the diagnosis or issue.

- Provides wholistic care that addresses the needs of diverse populations across the life span.

- Advocates for health care that is sensitive to the needs of healthcare consumers, with particular emphasis on the spiritual needs of diverse populations.

- Applies appropriate knowledge of major health problems and cultural diversity in implementing the plan of care.

- Applies available healthcare technologies to maximize access and optimize outcomes for healthcare consumers.

- Utilizes community and faith community resources and systems to implement the plan.

- Collaborates with healthcare providers from diverse backgrounds, spiritual leaders, caregivers, and volunteers to implement and integrate the plan.

- Accommodates different styles of communication used by healthcare consumers, families, and healthcare providers.

■ Integrates traditional and complementary healthcare practices as appropriate.

■ Implements the plan in a timely manner in accordance with healthcare consumer safety goals.

■ Promotes the person's capacity for the optimal level of participation and problem-solving, honoring the person's choices.

■ Documents implementation and any modifications, including changes or omissions, of the specified plan.

ADDITIONAL COMPETENCIES FOR THE GRADUATE-LEVEL PREPARED FAITH COMMUNITY NURSE AND THE ADVANCED PRACTICE REGISTERED NURSE

The graduate-level prepared faith community nurse or advanced practice registered nurse:

■ Facilitates utilization of systems in the faith community and other community resources when necessary to implement the plan.

■ Supports the development of interprofessional collaboration to implement the plan.

■ Incorporates new knowledge and strategies to initiate change in faith community nursing care practices if desired outcomes are not achieved.

■ Assumes responsibility for the safe and efficient implementation of the plan of care.

■ Uses advanced communication skills to promote interpersonal closeness between nurses and healthcare consumers, to provide a context for open discussion of the healthcare consumer's experiences, and to improve outcomes.

■ Implements the plan using principles and concepts of project or systems management.

■ Fosters organizational systems that support implementation of the plan.

■ Actively participates in the development and continuous improvement of systems that support the implementation of the plan.

Standard 5A. Coordination of Care

The faith community nurse coordinates care delivery.

COMPETENCIES

The faith community nurse:

- Coordinates implementation of a wholistic plan of care.

- Coordinates the health care of individuals across the life span using principles of interprofessional models of care delivery and case management.

- Organizes the components of the plan.

- Manages a healthcare consumer's care in order to maximize independence and quality of life.

- Assists the healthcare consumer to identify options for alternative care.

- Communicates with the healthcare consumer, family, and system during transitions in care.

- Advocates for the delivery of dignified and humane care by the interprofessional team.

- Documents the coordination of care.

ADDITIONAL COMPETENCIES FOR THE GRADUATE-LEVEL PREPARED FAITH COMMUNITY NURSE AND THE ADVANCED PRACTICE REGISTERED NURSE

The graduate-level prepared faith community nurse or advanced practice registered nurse:

- Provides leadership in the coordination of interprofessional health care for integrated delivery of healthcare consumer care services.

- Synthesizes data and information to prescribe necessary system and community support measures, including environmental modifications.

- Coordinates system and community resources that enhance delivery of care across continuums.

- Provides leadership in advocating for the delivery of dignified and humane care.

Standard 5B. Health Teaching and Health Promotion

The faith community nurse employs strategies to promote wholistic health, wellness, and a safe environment.

COMPETENCIES

The faith community nurse:

- Provides health teaching for individuals or groups that addresses such topics as healthy lifestyles, risk-reducing behaviors, developmental needs, activities of daily living, preventive self-care, and spiritual practices for health and healing.

- Uses health promotion and health teaching methods appropriate to the situation and the healthcare consumer's values, beliefs, health practices, developmental level, learning needs, readiness and ability to learn, language preference, spirituality, culture, and socioeconomic status.

- Seeks ongoing opportunities for feedback and evaluation of the effectiveness of the strategies used.

- Uses information technologies to communicate health promotion and disease prevention information to the healthcare consumer in a variety of settings.

- Provides healthcare consumers with information about intended effects and potential adverse effects of proposed therapies.

- Teaches activities that strengthen the body–mind–spirit connection, such as meditation, prayer, and guided imagery.

- Evaluates health information resources for use in faith community nursing for accuracy, readability, and comprehensibility by healthcare consumers, and compatibility with the healthcare consumers' spiritual beliefs and practices.

ADDITIONAL COMPETENCIES FOR THE GRADUATE-LEVEL PREPARED FAITH COMMUNITY NURSE AND THE ADVANCED PRACTICE REGISTERED NURSE

The graduate-level prepared faith community nurse or advanced practice registered nurse:

- Synthesizes empirical evidence on spiritual practices, risk behaviors, learning theories, behavioral change theories, motivational theories, epidemiology, and other related theories and frameworks when designing wholistic health information and healthcare consumer education.

- Conducts personalized health teaching and counseling considering comparative effectiveness research recommendations.

- Designs health information and healthcare consumer education appropriate to the healthcare consumer's spiritual beliefs and practices, cultural values and beliefs, developmental level, learning needs, readiness to learn, and readiness to experience new spiritual practices.

- Evaluates health information resources, such as the Internet, for accuracy, readability, and comprehensibility to help healthcare consumers to access quality health information that is compatible with their spiritual beliefs and practices.

- Engages faith-based organizations, consumer alliances, and advocacy groups, as appropriate, in health teaching and health promotion activities that are restorative, supportive, and promotive in nature.

- Provides anticipatory guidance to individuals, families, and groups in the faith communities to promote health and prevent or reduce the risk of health problems.

Standard 5C. Consultation

The faith community nurse provides consultation to facilitate understanding and influence the specified plan of care, enhance the abilities of others, and effect change.

COMPETENCIES

The faith community nurse:

- Initiates consultation with chaplains and spiritual leaders for resources, guidance, and support within the spiritual realm.

- Facilitates the effectiveness of a consultation by involving the healthcare consumer in decision-making and role negotiation.

- Consults with APRNs and other healthcare providers.

- Communicates consultation recommendations.

ADDITIONAL COMPETENCIES FOR THE GRADUATE-LEVEL PREPARED FAITH COMMUNITY NURSE AND THE ADVANCED PRACTICE REGISTERED NURSE

The graduate-level prepared faith community nurse or advanced practice registered nurse:

- Synthesizes spiritual practices, organizational structure, and beliefs of the faith group; clinical data; theoretical frameworks; and evidence when providing consultation.

- Facilitates the effectiveness of a consultation by involving the healthcare consumer or their designee in decision-making and negotiating role responsibilities for each member of the faith community.

- Communicates consultation recommendations effectively to influence the identified plan, facilitate understanding, enhance the work of the faith community team, and effect lasting change.

- Provides, structures, and maintains a safe therapeutic environment in collaboration with healthcare consumers, families, and other healthcare clinicians.

Standard 5D. Prescriptive Authority and Treatment

The advanced practice registered nurse uses prescriptive authority, procedures, referrals, treatments, and therapies in accordance with state and federal laws and regulations.

COMPETENCIES FOR THE ADVANCED PRACTICE REGISTERED NURSE

The advanced practice registered nurse:

- Prescribes evidence-based treatments, therapies, and procedures considering the healthcare consumer's comprehensive healthcare needs and spiritual needs, beliefs, and practices.

- Prescribes therapies, including those that strengthen the body–mind–spirit connection such as meditation, prayer, guided imagery, and various rituals of worship.

- Prescribes pharmacological agents according to a current knowledge of pharmacology and physiology.

- Prescribes specific pharmacological agents or treatments based on clinical indicators, the healthcare consumer's status and needs, and the results of diagnostic and laboratory tests.

- Evaluates therapeutic and potential adverse effects of pharmacological and nonpharmacological treatments.

- Provides healthcare consumers with information about intended effects and potential adverse effects of proposed prescriptive therapies.

- Provides information about costs and alternative treatments and procedures, as appropriate.

- Evaluates and incorporates complementary and alternative therapy into education and practice.

Standard 6. Evaluation

The faith community nurse evaluates progress toward attainment of outcomes.

COMPETENCIES

The faith community nurse:

- Conducts a wholistic, systematic, ongoing, and criterion-based evaluation of the outcomes in relation to the structures and processes prescribed by the plan and the indicated timeline.

- Collaborates with the healthcare consumer and others involved in the care or situation in the evaluative process.

- Evaluates, in partnership with the healthcare consumer, the effectiveness of the planned strategies in relation to the healthcare consumer's responses and attainment of expected outcomes.

- Uses ongoing assessment data to revise the diagnoses, the outcomes, the plan, and the plan's implementation as needed.

- Disseminates the results to the healthcare consumer and others involved in the care or situation, as appropriate, in accordance with state and federal laws and regulations.

- Participates in assessing and ensuring the responsible and appropriate use of interventions in order to minimize unwarranted or unwanted treatment and healthcare consumer suffering.

- Documents the results of the evaluation, including results from the faith or spiritual realm.

ADDITIONAL COMPETENCIES FOR THE GRADUATE-LEVEL PREPARED FAITH COMMUNITY NURSE AND THE ADVANCED PRACTICE REGISTERED NURSE

The graduate-level prepared faith community nurse or the advanced practice registered nurse:

- Evaluates the accuracy of the diagnosis and effectiveness of the interventions in relation to the healthcare consumer's attainment of expected outcomes.

- Uses spiritual assessment tools to identify the influence of the healthcare consumer's and family's views of health and healing on attainment of outcomes.

- Synthesizes the results of the evaluation analyses to determine the impact of the plan on the affected healthcare consumers, families, groups, faith communities and institutions, collegial networks, organizations, and geopolitical communities.

- Adapts the plan of care as well as policy and procedures of practice for the trajectory of treatment, when appropriate, based on evaluation of response by individuals and groups in faith communities.

- Uses the results of the evaluation to make or recommend process or structural changes, including policy, procedure, or protocol revision, as appropriate.

- Uses the results of the evaluation analyses to increase awareness beyond the individual faith community of the wholistic health benefits and spiritual care provided through faith community nursing.

Standards of Professional Performance for Faith Community Nursing

Standard 7. Ethics

The faith community nurse practices ethically.

COMPETENCIES

The faith community nurse:

- Uses *Code of Ethics for Nurses with Interpretive Statements* (ANA, 2001) to guide practice.

- Delivers care in a manner that preserves and protects the healthcare consumer's autonomy, dignity, rights, and spiritual beliefs and practices.

- Recognizes the centrality of the healthcare consumer and family as core members of any healthcare team.

- Upholds healthcare consumer confidentiality within religious, legal, and regulatory parameters.

- Assists healthcare consumers in self-determination and informed decision-making.

- Maintains a therapeutic and professional healthcare consumer–nurse relationship within appropriate professional role boundaries.

- Contributes to resolving ethical issues of healthcare consumers, colleagues, community groups, or systems, and other stakeholders.

- Takes appropriate action regarding instances of illegal, unethical, or inappropriate behavior that can endanger or jeopardize the best interests of the healthcare consumer or situation.

■ Speaks up as appropriate to question healthcare practice when necessary for safety and quality improvement.

■ Advocates for equitable healthcare consumer care.

■ Empowers healthcare consumers in developing skills for self-advocacy in support of their spiritual beliefs and practices.

■ Incorporates ethical and moral theories, principles, and models in processes of care planning and delivery.

■ Acknowledges and respects tenets of the faith and spiritual belief system of a healthcare consumer.

ADDITIONAL COMPETENCIES FOR THE GRADUATE-LEVEL PREPARED FAITH COMMUNITY NURSE AND THE ADVANCED PRACTICE REGISTERED NURSE

The graduate-level prepared faith community nurse or the advanced practice registered nurse:

■ Provides information on the risks, benefits, and outcomes of healthcare regimens to allow informed decision-making by the healthcare consumer, including informed consent and informed refusal.

■ Participates in interprofessional teams that address ethical risks, benefits, and outcomes of programs and decisions that affect health and healthcare delivery.

■ Mentors interprofessional teams in processes of ethical decision-making.

■ Advocates for equitable healthcare consumer care.

Standard 8. Education

The faith community nurse attains knowledge and competence that reflect current nursing practice.

COMPETENCIES

The faith community nurse:

- Participates in ongoing educational activities related to appropriate knowledge bases, professional issues, and spiritual care.

- Demonstrates a commitment to lifelong learning through self-reflection and inquiry to address learning and personal growth needs.

- Seeks experiences that reflect current practice to maintain knowledge, skills, abilities, and judgment in clinical practice or role performance for faith community nursing.

- Acquires knowledge and skills appropriate to the role, population, specialty of faith community nursing, setting, or situation.

- Seeks formal and independent learning experience to develop and maintain clinical, professional, and theological skills and knowledge.

- Identifies learning needs based on nursing knowledge, the various roles the nurse may assume, and the changing needs of the population.

- Participates in formal or informal consultations to address issues in nursing practice as an application of education and knowledge base.

- Shares educational findings, experiences, and ideas with peers.

- Contributes to a work environment conducive to the education of healthcare professionals.

- Maintains professional records that provide evidence of competence and lifelong learning.

ADDITIONAL COMPETENCIES FOR THE GRADUATE-LEVEL PREPARED FAITH COMMUNITY NURSE AND THE ADVANCED PRACTICE REGISTERED NURSE

The graduate-level prepared faith community nurse or the advanced practice registered nurse:

- Uses current healthcare research findings and other evidence to expand clinical and professional knowledge in order to better combine the two domains, nursing and spiritual care, into one practice role.

Standard 9. Evidence-Based Practice and Research

The faith community nurse integrates evidence and research findings into practice.

COMPETENCIES

The faith community nurse:

- Utilizes current evidence-based nursing knowledge, including research findings, to guide practice.

- Incorporates evidence when initiating changes in nursing practice.

- Participates, as appropriate to education level and position, in the formulation of evidence-based practice through research.

- Shares personal or third-party research findings with colleagues and peers.

ADDITIONAL COMPETENCIES FOR THE GRADUATE-LEVEL PREPARED FAITH COMMUNITY NURSE AND THE ADVANCED PRACTICE REGISTERED NURSE

The graduate-level prepared faith community nurse or the advanced practice registered nurse:

- Contributes to nursing knowledge by conducting or synthesizing research that discovers, examines, and evaluates knowledge, theories, criteria, and creative approaches to integrating spiritual care and nursing care in a faith community.

- Disseminates research findings through interdisciplinary activities such as presentations, publications, consultations, and journal clubs.

- Cultivates a climate of research and clinical inquiry.

Standard 10. Quality of Practice

The faith community nurse contributes to quality nursing practice.

COMPETENCIES

The faith community nurse:

- Demonstrates quality by documenting the application of the nursing process in a responsible, accountable, and ethical manner.

- Uses creativity, innovation in faith community nursing practice, and the resources of clergy, chaplains, hospice staff, and other colleagues to improve care delivery.

- Participates in quality improvement activities for faith community nursing. Such activities may include:

  - Identifying aspects of practice important for quality monitoring.

  - Using indicators to monitor quality and effectiveness of faith community nursing practice.

  - Collecting data to monitor quality and effectiveness of faith community nursing practice.

  - Analyzing quality data to identify opportunities for improving faith community nursing practice.

  - Formulating recommendations to improve faith community nursing practice or outcomes.

  - Implementing activities to enhance the quality of faith community nursing practice.

  - Developing, implementing, and evaluating policies, procedures, and guidelines to improve the quality of care.

  - Participating on and leading interprofessional teams to evaluate clinical care or health services.

  - Participating in and leading efforts to minimize costs and unnecessary duplication.

- Identifying problems that occur in day-to-day work routines in order to correct process inefficiencies.

- Analyzing factors related to quality, safety, and effectiveness.

- Analyzing organizational systems in the faith community for barriers to quality healthcare consumer outcomes.

- Implementing processes to remove or weaken barriers within the organizational systems in healthcare settings and the faith community.

- Participating in prayer, spiritual direction, and other intentional spiritual practices to enhance sustainability, personal growth, and skills as a spiritual care provider.

ADDITIONAL COMPETENCIES FOR THE GRADUATE-LEVEL PREPARED FAITH COMMUNITY NURSE AND THE ADVANCED PRACTICE REGISTERED NURSE

The graduate-level prepared faith community nurse or the advanced practice registered nurse:

- Provides leadership in the design and implementation of quality improvement activities.

- Designs innovations to effect change in practice and improve health outcomes.

- Evaluates the practice environment and quality of nursing care rendered in relation to existing evidence, identifying opportunities for the generation and use of research.

- Develops indicators to monitor quality and effectiveness of faith community nursing practice.

Standard 11. Communication

The faith community nurse communicates effectively in a variety of formats in all areas of practice.

COMPETENCIES

The faith community nurse:

- Assesses communication format preferences of healthcare consumers, families, and colleagues.

- Assesses his or her own communication skills in encounters with healthcare consumers, families, and colleagues.

- Seeks continuous improvement of his or her own communication and conflict-resolution skills.

- Conveys information to healthcare consumers, families, the interprofessional team, and others in communication formats that promote accuracy.

- Questions the rationale supporting routine approaches to care processes and decisions when they do not appear to be in the best interest of the healthcare consumer.

- Discloses observations or concerns related to hazards and errors in care or the practice environment to the appropriate level.

- Maintains communication with other providers to minimize risks associated with transfers and transition in care delivery.

- Contributes her or his own professional perspective in discussions with the interprofessional team.

Standard 12. Leadership

The faith community nurse demonstrates leadership in the professional practice setting and the profession.

COMPETENCIES

The faith community nurse:

- Oversees the nursing care given by others while retaining accountability for the quality of care given to the healthcare consumer.

- Abides by the vision, associated goals, and plan to implement and measure progress of an individual healthcare consumer or progress within the context of the healthcare organization.

- Demonstrates a commitment to continuous, lifelong learning, education, and spiritual growth for self and others.

- Mentors colleagues in relation to spirituality for the advancement of nursing practice, the profession, and quality health care.

- Treats colleagues with respect, trust, and dignity.

- Develops communication and conflict resolution skills.

- Participates in professional organizations.

- Communicates effectively with the healthcare consumer and colleagues.

- Seeks ways to advance nursing autonomy and accountability.

- Participates in efforts to influence healthcare policy involving healthcare consumers and the profession.

- Serves in key leadership roles in the faith community by participating on committees, councils, and health ministry administrative teams.

ADDITIONAL COMPETENCIES FOR THE GRADUATE-LEVEL PREPARED FAITH COMMUNITY NURSE AND THE ADVANCED PRACTICE REGISTERED NURSE

The graduate-level prepared faith community nurse or the advanced practice registered nurse:

- Influences decision-making bodies to improve the professional practice environment and healthcare consumer outcomes.

- Provides direction to enhance the effectiveness of the interprofessional team.

- Promotes advanced practice nursing and role development by interpreting its role for healthcare consumers, families, and others.

- Models expert practice to interprofessional team members and healthcare consumers.

- Mentors colleagues in the acquisition of clinical knowledge, skills, abilities, ethics, and judgment.

- Leads in enhancing the effectiveness of the interprofessional team.

- Promotes advancement of the profession through activities such as publishing, public speaking, and participation in professional organizations.

- Initiates revision of protocols or guidelines for community care to reflect evidence-based faith community nursing practice, to reflect the benefit of care management by faith community nurses, or to address emerging problems.

- Analyzes the economic, legal, regulatory, and political factors that influence healthcare delivery.

- Designs innovations to effect change in faith community nursing practice and improve the outcomes of wholistic health and healing.

Standard 13. Collaboration

The faith community nurse collaborates with the healthcare consumer, family, and others in the conduct of nursing practice.

COMPETENCIES

The faith community nurse:

- Partners with others to effect change and produce positive outcomes through the sharing of knowledge about the healthcare consumer and the situation.

- Communicates with the healthcare consumer, family, groups, spiritual leaders, hospital and hospice chaplains, and other healthcare providers regarding healthcare consumer care and the faith community nurse's role in the provision of that care.

- Promotes conflict management and engagement.

- Participates in consensus building or conflict resolution in the context of healthcare consumer care within faith community and healthcare settings.

- Applies group process and negotiation techniques with healthcare consumers and colleagues.

- Adheres to standards and applicable codes of conduct that govern behavior among peers and colleagues to create a work environment that promotes cooperation, respect, and trust.

- Cooperates in creating a documented plan focused on outcomes and decisions related to care and delivery of services that indicates communication with healthcare consumers, families, and others.

- Engages in teamwork and team-building processes.

- Documents referrals, including hospice and other provisions for continuity of care outside the faith community.

ADDITIONAL COMPETENCIES FOR THE GRADUATE-LEVEL PREPARED FAITH COMMUNITY NURSE AND THE ADVANCED PRACTICE REGISTERED NURSE

The graduate-level prepared faith community nurse or the advanced practice registered nurse:

- Partners with other disciplines to enhance healthcare consumer outcomes through interprofessional activities, such as education, consultation, management, technological development, or research opportunities.

- Invites the contribution of the healthcare consumer, family, and team members in order to achieve optimal outcomes.

- Leads in establishing, improving, and sustaining collaborative relationships to achieve safe, quality healthcare consumer care.

- Documents plan-of-care communications, rationales for plan-of-care changes, and collaborative discussions to improve healthcare consumer outcomes.

- Participates on interprofessional teams that contribute to role development and, directly or indirectly, advance nursing practice and health services.

Standard 14. Professional Practice Evaluation

The faith community nurse evaluates his or her own nursing practice in relation to professional practice standards and guidelines, relevant statutes, rules, and regulations.

COMPETENCIES

The faith community nurse's practice reflects the application of knowledge of current practice standards, guidelines, statutes, rules, and regulations.

The faith community nurse:

- Provides age-appropriate and developmentally appropriate care in a spiritually, culturally, and ethnically sensitive manner.

- Engages in self-evaluation of practice regularly, identifying areas of strength as well as areas in which professional development would be beneficial.

- Obtains informal feedback regarding her or his own spiritual care and nursing practice from healthcare consumers, peers, spiritual leaders, health committee members, faith community volunteers, professional colleagues, and others.

- Participates in systematic formal review, as appropriate.

- Takes action to achieve goals identified during the evaluation process.

- Provides evidence for practice decisions and actions as part of the informal and formal evaluation processes.

- Interacts with peers and colleagues to enhance her or his own professional nursing practice or role performance.

- Provides peers with formal or informal constructive feedback regarding their practice or role performance.

ADDITIONAL COMPETENCIES FOR THE GRADUATE-LEVEL PREPARED FAITH COMMUNITY NURSE AND THE ADVANCED PRACTICE REGISTERED NURSE

The graduate-level prepared faith community nurse or the advanced practice registered nurse:

- Engages in a formal process seeking feedback regarding her or his own practice from healthcare consumers, peers, professional colleagues, and others.

Standard 15. Resource Utilization

The faith community nurse utilizes appropriate resources to plan and provide nursing services that are safe, effective, and financially responsible.

COMPETENCIES

The faith community nurse:

- Assesses individual healthcare consumer care needs and resources available to achieve desired outcomes.

- Identifies healthcare consumer care needs, potential for harm, complexity of the task, and desired outcome when considering resource allocation.

- Delegates elements of care to appropriate healthcare workers in accordance with any applicable legal or policy parameters or principles.

- Identifies the evidence when evaluating resources.

- Advocates for resources, including technology, that enhance nursing practice.

- Modifies practice when necessary to promote a positive interface between healthcare consumers, care providers, and technology.

- Assists the healthcare consumer and family in identifying and securing appropriate and available resources to address health and spiritually related needs across the healthcare continuum.

- Assists the healthcare consumer and family in factoring costs, risks, and benefits in decisions about treatment and care.

- Develops innovative solutions and applies strategies to obtain appropriate resources for faith community nursing care.

ADDITIONAL COMPETENCIES FOR THE GRADUATE-LEVEL PREPARED FAITH COMMUNITY NURSE AND THE ADVANCED PRACTICE REGISTERED NURSE

The graduate-level prepared faith community nurse or the advanced practice registered nurse:

- Utilizes organizational and community resources to formulate interprofessional plans of care.

- Formulates innovative solutions for healthcare consumer care problems that utilize resources effectively and maintain quality.

- Designs evaluation strategies that demonstrate cost-effectiveness, cost–benefit, and efficiency factors associated with nursing practice.

Standard 16. Environmental Health

The faith community nurse practices in an environmentally safe and healthy manner.

COMPETENCIES

The faith community nurse:

- Attains knowledge of environmental health concepts, such as implementation of environmental health strategies.

- Promotes a practice environment that reduces environmental health risks for workers and healthcare consumers.

- Assesses the practice environment for such factors as sound, odor, noise, and light that threaten health.

- Advocates for the judicious and appropriate use of products in health care.

- Communicates environmental health risks and exposure reduction strategies to healthcare consumers, families, colleagues, faith communities, and broader communities.

- Utilizes scientific evidence to determine if a product or treatment is an environmental threat.

- Participates in strategies to promote healthy communities.

- Addresses environmental health risks in the home, workplace, faith community, and healthcare setting.

- Advocates for environmental health and social justice, including a commitment to the health of vulnerable populations.

ADDITIONAL COMPETENCIES FOR THE GRADUATE-LEVEL PREPARED FAITH COMMUNITY NURSE AND THE ADVANCED PRACTICE REGISTERED NURSE

The graduate-level prepared faith community nurse or the advanced practice registered nurse:

- Creates partnerships that promote sustainable environmental health policies and conditions.

- Analyzes the impact of social, political, and economic influences on the environment and human health exposures.

- Critically evaluates the manner in which environmental health issues are presented by the popular media.

- Advocates for implementation of environmental principles for nursing practice.

- Identifies patterns of comorbidities among family and community members suggesting environmental etiologies.

Glossary

Assessment. A systematic, dynamic process by which a faith community registered nurse, through interaction with the healthcare consumer, family, groups, communities, populations, spiritual leaders, and healthcare providers, collects and analyzes data. In addition to spiritual dimensions, assessment by the faith community registered nurse may include the following dimensions: physical, psychological, sociocultural, cognitive, functional abilities, developmental, economic, environmental, and lifestyle.

Caregiver. A person who provides direct care for another, such as a child, a dependent adult, or a person with a disability, chronic illness, or spiritual distress.

Code of ethics. A succinct list of provisions that makes explicit the primary goals, values, and obligations of the profession.

Competency. An expected and measurable level of nursing performance that integrates knowledge, skills, abilities, and judgment and that is based on established scientific knowledge and expectations for nursing practice.

Continuity of care. An interdisciplinary process that includes healthcare consumers, families, significant others, and appropriate members of a faith community in the development of a coordinated plan of care. This process facilitates the healthcare consumer's transition between settings and healthcare providers, based on changing needs and available resources.

Diagnosis. A clinical judgment about the healthcare consumer's response to actual, perceived, or potential health concerns or needs. The diagnosis provides the basis for determining a plan to achieve desired outcomes, to establish priorities, and to develop a plan of action with the healthcare consumer. Faith community registered nurses utilize nursing diagnoses or medical diagnoses depending on their education, clinical preparation, and legal authority.

Disease. A biological or psychosocial disorder of structure or function in a healthcare consumer, especially a disorder that produces specific signs or symptoms or that affects a specific part of the body, mind, or spirit.

Documentation. The recording of the assessment, plan of care, interventions, and evaluation of outcomes in a retrievable format that is confidential and secure for the healthcare consumer to facilitate continuity in meeting desired health outcomes.

Environment. The atmosphere, milieu, or conditions in which an individual lives, works, plays, or carries out his or her faith practices.

Evaluation. The process of determining the progress toward attainment of expected outcomes and the satisfaction of the healthcare consumer with those outcomes for the purpose of modifying the plan. Outcomes include the effectiveness of care, when addressing one's own practice.

Evidence-based practice. A process founded on the collection, interpretation, and integration of valid, important, and applicable healthcare consumer reported, clinician-observed, and research-derived evidence. The best available evidence, moderated by healthcare consumer circumstances and preferences, is applied to improve the quality of clinical judgments.

Faith community. An organization of groups, families, and individuals who share common values, beliefs, religious doctrine, and faith practices that influence their lives, generally in the setting of a church, synagogue, temple, mosque or faith-based agency, and that functions as a healthcare consumer system, providing a setting for faith community nursing.

Faith community nurse (FCN). A registered professional nurse who is actively licensed in a given state and who serves as a member of the staff of a faith community. The FCN promotes health as wholeness of the faith community, its groups, families, and individual members through the practice of nursing as defined by that state's nurse practice act in the jurisdiction in which the FCN practices and the standards of practice set forth in this document.

Faith community nursing. The specialized practice of professional nursing that focuses on the intentional care of the spirit as well as on the promotion of wholistic health and prevention or minimization of illness within the context of a faith community.

Faith group. A specific denomination or sect within a faith tradition.

Family. Family of origin or significant others as identified by a healthcare consumer, who may refer to some or all of the members of a faith community as part of their family.

Group. A number of people sharing something in common, such as an interest, activity, or spiritual beliefs and practices.

Healing. The process of integrating the body, mind, and spirit to bring about wholeness, health, and a sense of spiritual well-being, although the healthcare consumer's disease may not be cured.

Health. The experience of wholeness, salvation, or shalom. The integration of the spiritual, physical, psychological, emotional, and social aspects of the healthcare consumer to create a sense of harmony with self, others, the environment, and a higher power. Health may be experienced in the presence or absence of disease or injury.

Healthcare consumer. The person, client, family, group, community, or population who is the focus of attention and to whom the registered nurse is providing services as sanctioned by the state regulatory bodies. The term *healthcare consumer* is used to provide consistency and brevity, bearing in mind that other terms, such as *client, individual, family, groups, community,* or *population,* might be better choices in some instances.

- When the healthcare consumer is an individual, the focus is on the health state, problems, or needs of the individual.

- When the healthcare consumer is a family or group, the focus is on the health of the unit as a whole or the reciprocal effects of the individual's health on the other members of the unit.

- When the healthcare consumer is a community or population, the focus is on personal and environmental health and the health risks of the community or population.

Healthcare providers. Individuals with special expertise who provide healthcare services or assistance to healthcare consumers. They may include nurses, physicians, spiritual leaders, psychologists, social workers, nutritionists/dietitians, and various therapists.

Health ministry. The promotion of health and healing as part of the mission and service of a faith community to its members and the community it serves.

Health promotion. Activities and interventions that healthcare consumers undertake to achieve desired health outcomes. Health promotion outcomes may be primary (the prevention of disease and injury); secondary (the early detection and appropriate intervention in illness or brokenness); or tertiary (the promotion of wholeness and sense of well-being when curing may not occur).

Illness. The subjective experience of discomfort, brokenness; the disintegration of body, mind, spirit; disharmony with others, the environment, or a higher power.

Implementation. Activities such as teaching, monitoring, providing, praying, leading meditation, counseling, delegating, and coordinating. Carrying out of a plan of action in a spiritual, caring relationship that provides the information, skills, motivation, spiritual or faith tradition rituals, and resources necessary to empower the healthcare consumer to achieve desired health outcomes.

Interprofessional. Reliant on overlapping knowledge, skills, and abilities of each team member and discipline, resulting in synergistic effects where outcomes are enhanced and more comprehensive than the simple aggregation of any team member's individual efforts.

Patient. See *Healthcare consumer.*

Peer review/evaluation. A collegial, systematic, and periodic process by which faith community nurses are held accountable for their practice and that fosters the refinement of one's knowledge, skills, and decision-making.

Plan. A comprehensive outline of the components that need to be completed to attain mutually identified and expected healthcare consumer outcomes.

Quality of care. The degree to which health services for healthcare consumers, families, groups, communities, or populations increase the likelihood of desired outcomes and are consistent with current professional knowledge.

Registered nurse (RN). An individual registered or licensed by a state, commonwealth, territory, government, or other regulatory body to practice as a registered nurse.

Restorative practices. Nursing interventions that mitigate the impact of illness or disease.

Scope of nursing practice. The description of the *who, what, where, when, why,* and *how* of nursing practice that addresses the range of nursing practice activities common to all registered nurses. When considered in conjunction with the Standards of Professional Nursing Practice and the Code of Ethics for Nurses, comprehensively describes the competent level of nursing common to all registered nurses.

Self-care. Actions a faith community, group, family, or individual take to attain desired wholistic health outcomes when they possess the requisite knowledge, skills, ability, resources, motivation, encouragement, and support.

Spiritual care. The practical expression of presence, guidance, and interventions, individual or communal, to support, nurture, or encourage an individual's or group's ability to achieve wholeness; health; personal, spiritual, and social well-being; integration of body, mind, and spirit; and a sense of connection to self, others, and a higher power.

Spiritual leader. An individual recognized and authorized by a faith community, such as a clergyperson (pastor, priest, rabbi, shaman), chaplain, or lay minister, who guides and inspires others in the study and nurture of their spiritual beliefs and application of spiritual practices.

Standard. An authoritative statement defined and promoted by the profession by which the quality of practice, service, or education can be evaluated.

Supportive practices. Nursing interventions that are oriented toward modification of relationships or the environment to support health.

Transitional care. Actions of faith community nurses and other healthcare providers designed to ensure the coordination and continuity of health care for healthcare consumers during movement between hospitals, sub-acute and post-acute nursing facilities, the healthcare consumer's home, primary and specialty care offices, and long-term care facilities as their condition and care needs change during the course of a chronic or acute illness.

Well-being. An individual's perception of her or his own wholistic health.

Wholistic. Based on an understanding that a healthcare consumer is an interconnected unity and that physical, mental, social, environmental, and spiritual factors need to be included in any interventions. The whole system, whether referring to a human being or a faith community, is greater than the sum of its parts. The preferred term when referring to the type of care provided by a faith community nurse.

The content in this appendix is not current and is of historical significance only.

References and Bibliography

American Nurses Association. (2001). *Code of ethics for nurses with interpretive statements*. Washington, DC: Nursesbooks.org.

American Nurses Association. (2010a). *Nursing: Scope and standards of practice, second edition*. Silver Spring, MD: Nursesbooks.org.

American Nurses Association. (2010b). *Nursing's social policy statement: The essence of the profession*. Silver Spring, MD: Nursesbooks.org.

Brown, A. R., Coppola, P., Giacona, M., Petriches, A., & Stockwell, M. A. (2009). Faith community nursing demonstrates good stewardship of community benefit dollars through cost savings and cost avoidance. *Family and Community Health, 32*(4), 330–338. doi.10.1097/FCH.0b013e3181b91f93

Catanzaro, A. M., Meador, K. G., Koenig, H. G., Kuchibhatla, M., & Clipp, E. C. (2007). Congregational health ministries: A national study of pastors' views. *Public Health Nursing, 24*(1), 6–17. doi: 10.1111/j.1525-1446.2006.00602.x

Chase-Ziolek, M. (2005). *Health, healing, and wholeness: Engaging congregations in ministries of health*. Cleveland, OH: Pilgrim Press.

Chase-Ziolek, M., & Iris, M. (2002). Nurses' perspectives on the distinctive aspects of providing nursing care in a congregational setting. *Journal of Community Health Nursing, 19*(3), 173–186.

Coleman, E. A., & Boult, C. E. (2003). Improving the quality of transitional care for persons with complex care needs. *Journal of the American Geriatrics Society, 51*(4), 556–557.

Donahue, M. P. (1996). *Nursing, the finest art: An illustrated history* (2nd ed.). St. Louis, MO: Mosby.

Dunn, H. L. (1959). High-level wellness for man and society. *Journal of Public Health, 49*(6), 786–792.

Dyess, S., Chase, S. K, & Newlin, K. (2010). State of research for faith community nursing 2009. *Journal of Religion and Health, 49*(2), 188–199.

Health Ministries Association and American Nurses Association. (1998). *Scope and standards of parish nursing practice.* Washington, DC: American Nurses Publishing.

Hickman, J. S. (2006). *Faith community nursing.* Philadelphia: Lippincott, Williams and Wilkins.

Institute of Medicine. (2010). *The future of nursing: Leading change, advancing health.* Washington, DC: National Academy of Sciences.

Koenig, H. G., McCullough, M. E., & Larson, D. B. (2001). *The handbook of religion and health.* Oxford, England: Oxford University Press.

Levin, J. (2002). *God, faith, and health: Exploring the spirituality-healing connection.* New York, NY: John Wiley and Sons.

Mayernik, D., Resick, L. K., Skomo, M. L., & Mandock, K. (2010). Parish nurse-initiated interdisciplinary mobile health care delivery project. *Journal of Obstetric, Gynecologic, and Neonatal Nursing, 39*(2), 227–234.

North American Nursing Diagnosis Association (NANDA). (2009). *Nursing diagnoses: Definitions and classification 2008–2009.* Philadelphia: NANDA International.

Puchalski, C. M., & Ferrell, B. (2010). *Making health care whole: Integrating spirituality into patient care.* West Conshohocken, PA: Templeton Press.

Rethemeyer, A., & Wehling, B. A. (2004). How are we doing? Measuring the effectiveness of parish nursing. *Journal of Christian Nursing, 21*(2), 10–12.

Smucker, C. J., & Weinberg, L. (2009). *Faith community nursing: Developing a quality practice.* Silver Spring, MD: Nursesbooks.org.

Solari-Twadell, P. A., & Hackbarth, D. P. (2010). Evidence for a new paradigm of the ministry of parish nursing practice using the nursing intervention classification system. *Nursing Outlook, 58*(2), 69–75.

Weis, D., Schank, M., Coenen, A., & Matheus, R. (2002). Parish nurse practice with client aggregates. *Journal of Community Health Nursing, 19*(2), 105–113.

The content in this appendix is not current and is of historical significance only.

Appendix B
Historic Milestones in Faith Community Nursing in the United States

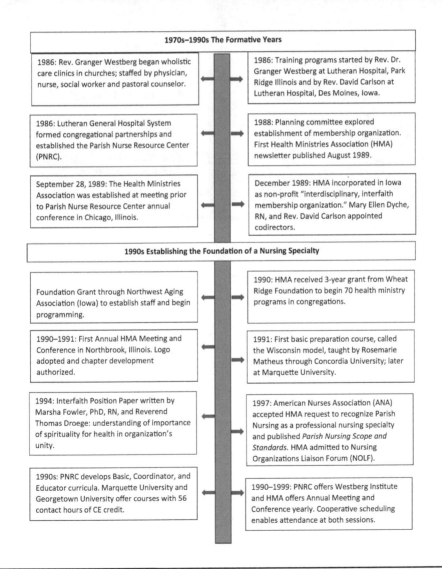

1970s–1990s The Formative Years

1986: Rev. Granger Westberg began wholistic care clinics in churches; staffed by physician, nurse, social worker and pastoral counselor.

1986: Training programs started by Rev. Dr. Granger Westberg at Lutheran Hospital, Park Ridge Illinois and by Rev. David Carlson at Lutheran Hospital, Des Moines, Iowa.

1986: Lutheran General Hospital System formed congregational partnerships and established the Parish Nurse Resource Center (PNRC).

1988: Planning committee explored establishment of membership organization. First Health Ministries Association (HMA) newsletter published August 1989.

September 28, 1989: The Health Ministries Association was established at meeting prior to Parish Nurse Resource Center annual conference in Chicago, Illinois.

December 1989: HMA incorporated in Iowa as non-profit "interdisciplinary, interfaith membership organization." Mary Ellen Dyche, RN, and Rev. David Carlson appointed codirectors.

1990s Establishing the Foundation of a Nursing Specialty

Foundation Grant through Northwest Aging Association (Iowa) to establish staff and begin programming.

1990: HMA received 3-year grant from Wheat Ridge Foundation to begin 70 health ministry programs in congregations.

1990–1991: First Annual HMA Meeting and Conference in Northbrook, Illinois. Logo adopted and chapter development authorized.

1991: First basic preparation course, called the Wisconsin model, taught by Rosemarie Matheus through Concordia University; later at Marquette University.

1994: Interfaith Position Paper written by Marsha Fowler, PhD, RN, and Reverend Thomas Droege: understanding of importance of spirituality for health in organization's unity.

1997: American Nurses Association (ANA) accepted HMA request to recognize Parish Nursing as a professional nursing specialty and published *Parish Nursing Scope and Standards*. HMA admitted to Nursing Organizations Liaison Forum (NOLF).

1990s: PNRC develops Basic, Coordinator, and Educator curricula. Marquette University and Georgetown University offer courses with 56 contact hours of CE credit.

1990–1999: PNRC offers Westberg Institute and HMA offers Annual Meeting and Conference yearly. Cooperative scheduling enables attendance at both sessions.

2000s: Moving Forward Into the Future

2001: PNRC relocated to Deaconess Foundation, St. Louis, Missouri; changes name to International Parish Nurse Resource Center (IPNRC); sponsors 16th Annual Westberg Parish Nurse Symposium.

2002: HMA inaugurates the Wilkerson-Droege Award in honor of Sister June Wilkerson and Reverend Thomas Droege.

2005: Revision of *Parish Nursing Scope and Standards of Practice*. Title changed to *Faith Community Nursing Scope and Standards of Practice*

2007: HMA begins initial work with American Nurses Credentialing Center (ANCC) to develop formal recognition process for faith community nurses.

2009: HMA 20th anniversary year. Four Regional Educational Conferences held instead of Annual Conference.

2010: First HMA National Summit held in Burlingame, California. White paper *Now More Than Ever* published through grant support of Health and Human Services Office on Women's Health, Washington, DC.

2011: IPNRC moved to the Church Health Center in Memphis, Tennessee; celebrated the 25th anniversary of the Westberg Symposium.

2011: HMA establishes the Westberg Faith Community Nursing Leadership Award. HMA published *Health Minister Guidelines*. Second National Summit—Mobilizing Health Ministry for the 21st Century.

2012: *Faith Community Nursing Scope and Standards of Practice, 2nd Edition*, revised and published. National workshops on scope and standards presented in nine states.

2012: Agreement signed June 2012 between HMA and ANCC to begin development of Certification by Portfolio in Faith Community Nursing.

2014: ANCC offers Certification by Portfolio in Faith Community Nursing.

http://nursecredentialing.org/FaithCommunityNursing

2015: HMA establishes Faith Community Nursing Society. Recognizes nurses who have achieved certification by portfolio in faith community nursing.

2016: IPNRC name changed to Westberg Institute for Faith Community Nursing.

2016 2017: Collaborative process by ANA and HMA for revision of *Faith Community Nursing Scope and Standards of Practice, 3rd Edition*.
2017: ANA Board of Directors approves HMA as an Organizational Affiliate.

Index

Entries with (2012) indicate an entry from *Faith Community Nursing: Scope and Standards of Practice, 2nd Edition*, reproduced in the Appendix. That information is not current, and is included for its reference and historical value only.

resource utilization competencies,
79–80
(2012), 160–161
scope, 1
Advocacy, 3, 13–14, 25
defined, 83
Advocacy for patients and families, 2,
17, 20, 23–24, 34, 38
health teaching and health promotion
and, 59, 60
Advocate Health Care, 7, 28
Alternative medicine, 7
American Association of Colleges of
Nursing (AACN), 29
American Nurses Association (ANA)
*Code of Ethics for Nurses With
Interpretive Statements*, 4, 13,
15–24, 63, 78
*Faith Community Nursing: Scope and
Standards of Practice*, 4, 8, 10, 25,
78
American Nurses Credentialing Center
(ANCC), 9
American Psychiatric Association (APA),
38
Assessment, 9, 10, 12, 17, 18, 34, 35, 37
competencies for, 45–47, 49, 52, 53,
61
data, 45–46, 48
defined, 83
diagnosis and, 48, 49, 61
evaluation and, 61
planning and, 52, 53
standard of practice, 45–47
(2012) 130–131
Associate faith community leader, 20,
21
Automated external defibrillator (AED),
41
Autonomy of nurses in FCN practice, 15,
18, 26, 63, 71
defined, 83

B

*Baccalaureate Degree in Nursing as
Minimal Preparation for Professional
Practice, The*, 29

Behavioral health, 38
defined, 83
Benefits and costs. *See* Cost control
Biomedical ethics, principles of, 15
Body of knowledge in FCN practice, 28.
See also Evidence-based practice
(EBP); Knowledge, skills, abilities,
and judgment in FCN practice

C

Cardiopulmonary resuscitation (CPR), 41
Care
intentional, 1, 3, 4, 10
nursing, 4–5, 7, 10, 12, 27, 31, 39,
55, 71, 75, 76
recipients. *See* Healthcare consumers
self-care, 4, 41–42, 57, 64
spiritual, 2, 10–13, 25, 27, 28, 29,
32, 35, 38, 62, 73, 75
for stranger, 5
Care coordination. *See* Coordination of
care
Caregiver
defined, 84
Caring
defined, 84
Centers for Disease Control and
Prevention (CDC), 23
Certification
defined, 84
Certification and credentialing, 9, 26,
30, 43, 71, 76, 77
competencies for, 71, 76, 77
Certification by Portfolio in Faith
Community Nursing, 9
Certified nurse-midwife (CNM), 26
Certified nurse practitioner (CNP), 26, 27
Certified registered nurse anesthetist
(CRNA), 26, 27
Charity hospitals, 5
Church Health Center, 28
Churches, role in healing, 6
CINAHL, 21
Clients. *See* Healthcare consumers
Clinical Care Classification System (CCC),
11
Clinical nurse specialist (CNS), 26, 27

Code of ethics (nursing)
defined, 84
Code of Ethics for Nurses with Interpretive Statements and faith community
nursing practice, 13, 14, 63, 78
accountability and responsibility for
practice (Provision 4), 18–19
advocacy for the patient (Provision 3),
17–18
collaboration with the public and health
professionals (Provision 8), 22–23
commitment to the patient
(Provision 2), 16–17
duties to self and others (Provision 5),
19–20
exemplars, 15–24
nursing profession advancement
(Provision 7), 21–22
nursing professional integrity
and values and social justice
(Provision 9), 23–24
respect for the individual (Provision 1),
15–16
work settings and care environment
contributions (Provision 6), 20–21
Collaboration, 35
competencies for, 29, 54, 59, 69–79
defined, 84
health teaching and health promotion
and, 59
implementation and, 54
interprofessional, 29
standard of professional performance,
69–70
(2012), 156–157
Commitment to profession, 14, 16, 20,
31–32
Communication, 21, 23, 25, 31
assessment and, 45
collaboration and, 70
competencies for, 45, 48, 54, 67–68,
70
culturally congruent practice and, 65
diagnosis and, 48
implementation and, 54
standard of professional performance,
67–68
(2012), 153

Community, 4
Compassionate listening, 3
Compensation, 40–41
Competence in faith community nursing
practice, 19, 31, 73
defined, 31
Competency(ies) for faith community
nursing practice, 31, 43. *See also*
Advanced practice registered nurse
(APRN)/Advanced practice faith
community nurse; Graduate-level
prepared faith community nurse;
Specific standards
assessment, 45–47
(2012), 130–131
collaboration, 69–79
(2012), 156–157
communication, 67–68
(2012), 153
consultation (2012), 142
coordination of care, 57–58
(2012), 139
culturally congruent practice, 65–66
defined, 84
diagnosis, 48–49
(2012), 133
education, 73
(2012), 148–149
environmental health, 81–82
(2012), 162–163
ethics, 63–64
(2012), 146–147
evaluation, 61–62
(2012), 144–145
evidence-based practice and research,
74–75
(2012), 150
health teaching and health promotion,
59–60
(2012), 140–141
implementation, 54–56
(2012), 137–138
leadership, 71–72
(2012), 154–155
outcomes identification, 50–51
(2012), 133–134
planning, 52–53
(2012), 135–136

prescriptive authority and treatment (2012), 143

professional practice evaluation, 78
  (2012), 158–159

quality of practice, 76–77
  (2012), 151–152

resource utilization, 79–80
  (2012), 160–161

Confidentiality, 17, 18, 19, 21, 39, 40. *See also* Ethics; Privacy
  collaboration and, 69
  defined, 84
  ethics and, 64

Consultation, 27
  collaboration and, 70
  competencies for, 55, 56, 73, 75
  education and, 73
  evidence-based practice and research and, 75
  implementation and, 55, 56
  standards of practice, (2012), 142

Continuing education (CE) course, 8, 23, 28–29, 32, 71, 73. *See also* Education

Continuity of care, 37, 67
  coordination of care and, 57
  defined, 84

Coordination of care, 34
  competencies for, 50, 57–58
  outcomes identification and, 50
  standard of practice, 57–58
  (2012), 139

Costs and financial issues, 40. *See also* Resource utilization
  competencies, 50, 51, 52, 79
  cost control, 40
  outcome identification and, 50, 51
  planning and, 52
  resource utilization and, 79

Credentialing. *See* Certification and credentialing

Critical thinking, analysis, and synthesis, 26, 31, 39, 54. *See also* Evidence-based practice (EBP); Knowledge, skills, abilities, and judgment in FCN practice; Nursing process
  evidence-based practice and research and, 74

implementation and, 54
planning and, 53

Cultural competence, 24–25. *See also* Culturally congruent practice

Cultural knowledge
  defined, 85

Cultural skills
  defined, 85

Culturally congruent practice, 15–16, 24–25
  competencies for, 65–66
  standard of professional performance, 65–66

Curriculum, 4, 28

D

Databases, 33, 75

Data and information
  assessment data, 46, 48,
  competencies for, 45, 46, 48, 54, 56, 58, 61, 62, 76, 77
  data collection, 32, 39, 42
  evaluation data, 61, 62

Deacon, 6–7, 27

Decision-making, 14, 15, 16, 21, 29, 39
  competencies for, 48, 50, 55, 64, 65, 66, 77, 79
  culturally congruent practice and, 65, 66
  ethics and, 63, 64
  implementation and, 55
  leadership and, 72
  outcomes identification and, 50
  quality of practice and, 77

Delegation
  competencies for, 54, 71, 79
  defined, 85

Descriptive studies, 32

Diagnosis, 10
  competencies for, 48–49, 75
  defined, 85
  evidence-based practice and research and, 75
  standard of practice, 48–49
  (2012), 132

Diakonas, 6

Disease
  defined, 85
Documentation, 33, 39
  collaboration and, 70
  competencies for, 46, 48, 50, 53, 54,
    57, 61, 69, 70, 76
  defined, 85
Dunn, Halbert, 7

E

Economic controls. *See* Cost control
Ecosystem
  defined, 85
Education of faith community nurses,
    8, 9, 10, 19–20, 25–26. *See also*
    Advanced practice registered nurse
    (APRN)/Advanced practice faith
    community nurse
  advanced practice registered nurse,
    26–27
  approaches towards, 28–29
  collaboration and, 70
  competencies for, 26–31, 66, 70, 71
    73, 80
  culturally congruent practice and,
    66
  graduate-level-prepared RN, 26
  health teaching and health promotion
    and, 80
  leadership and, 71
  ongoing education and competence,
    31
  spiritual preparation, 29–30
  standard of professional performance,
    73
  (2012), 148–149
Education of patients and families, 3, 5,
    37, 39. *See also* Health teaching
    and health promotion
Electronic health record (EHR) system,
    11, 39
Emergency actions, 41
Environment
  defined, 85
Environmental health
  competencies for, 81–82
  defined, 86

standard of professional performance,
    81–82
  (2012), 162–163
*Essentials of Baccalaureate Education
  for Professional Nursing Practice*,
    10
Ethical decision-making, 15. *See also*
    Decision-making; Ethics; *Code of
    Ethics with Interpretive Statements*
    for faith community nurses
Ethical healthcare, 13
Ethics, 13–24
  competencies for, 63–64, 78
  professional practice evaluation and, 78
  standard of professional performance,
    63–64
  (2012), 146–147
Evaluation
  competencies for, 61–62
  defined, 86
  standard of practice, 61–62
  (2012), 144–145
Evidence-based practice (EBP), 2, 41.
    See also Research
  competencies for, 50, 60, 74–75
  defined, 86
  health teaching and health promotion
    and, 60
  outcomes identification and, 50
  standard of professional performance,
    74–75
  (2012), 150
Expected outcomes. *See also* Outcomes
    identification
  defined, 86
  diagnosis and, 48
Experiential learning, 30

F

Facilitation Center for Nursing
    Classification and Clinical
    Effectiveness, 10
Faith community, 2, 6
  defined, 86
Faith community nurses (FCNs)
  assessment competencies, 45–46
  collaboration competencies, 69

communication competencies, 67
coordination of care competencies, 57
culturally congruent practice competencies, 65–66
defined, 86
development of expected role, 5
diagnosis competencies, 48
education competencies, 25–26, 73
and elderly couple, 16–17
environmental health competencies, 81
ethics competencies, 63–64
evaluation competencies, 61
evidence-based practice and research competencies, 74
health teaching and health promotion competencies, 59
implementation competencies, 54
leadership competencies, 71
outcomes identification competencies, 50
planning competencies, 52–53
professional practice evaluation competencies, 78
quality of practice competencies, 76
resource utilization competencies, 79
scope of practice, 1–43
and settings, 5
standards of practice, 45–62
standards of professional performance, 63–82
Faith community nursing
activities, 36
core values of, 4
curriculum, 4
defined, 1–2, 86
description of the scope, 1
distinguishing tenets of, 3
educational preparation for, 25–32
ethics in, 13–24
evolution of, 6–9
foundations of practice, 4
practice settings, 4–6
professional trends and issues in, 33–42
research and, 32–33
specialty of, 2–3

Faith Community Nursing: Scope and Standards of Practice, 8, 9
Faith denominations, 28, 32
Faith group, 14, 27
defined, 86
Family, 22, 35
assessment and, 46
caregivers, 16
collaboration and, 69, 70
coordination of care and, 57
culturally congruent practice and, 65
defined, 87
diagnosis and, 48
education and, 73
environmental health and, 82
ethics and, 63
evaluation and, 61
implementation and, 54
outcomes identification and, 50
planning and, 52
Feedback, 59, 69, 78
Financial issues. *See Costs and financial issues.*
Folk health care systems, 16
Folk medicine practices, 24
Formal learning, 31

G

Generic care systems, 24
Graduate courses, 29
Graduate-level-prepared faith community nurse
assessment competencies, 46
collaboration competencies, 70
communication competencies, 68
coordination of care competencies, 57–58
culturally congruent practice competencies, 66
diagnosis competencies, 48
environmental health competencies, 82
ethics competencies, 64
evaluation competencies, 61–62
evidence-based practice and research competencies, 74–75
health teaching and health promotion competencies, 60

implementation competencies, 55
leadership competencies, 72
outcomes identification competencies, 51
planning competencies, 52
quality of practice competencies, 76–77
resource allocation competencies, 79–80
Graduate-level-prepared registered nurse, 26
defined, 87
Grant support, 8
Group
defined, 87
Guidelines in faith community nursing
assessment and, 46
ethics and, 63
quality of practice and, 76, 77

H

Healing, 4
defined, 87
Health
defined, 87
Health information, accuracy of, 42
Health Insurance Portability and Accountability Act of 1996 (HIPAA), 20, 21
Health Ministries Association (HMA), 3, 4, 7, 8, 9, 13, 23, 24, 28, 30, 32, 41, 42
Health ministry
defined, 87
Health promotion
defined, 87
Health teaching and health promotion, 3, 7, 8, 12, 22, 23, 27, 35, 36
competencies for, 41–42, 59–60
and self-care, 41–42
standard of practice, 59–60
(2012), 140–141
Healthcare consumers, 3, 5, 35. *See also* Patients.
collaboration and, 70
communication and, 67
coordination of care and, 57

culturally congruent practice and, 65, 66
defined, 2, 87–88
diagnosis and, 48
environmental health and, 81
ethics and, 63, 64
evidence-based practice and research and, 75
health teaching and promotion and, 59, 60
implementation and, 54, 56
leadership and, 72
planning and, 53
professional practice evaluation and, 78
quality of practice and, 77
resource utilization and, 79
spiritual care and, 10
Healthcare providers, 20, 31, 34, 35
collaboration and, 69
defined, 88
outcomes identification and, 50
Healthcare-system-based models, 37
Healthy People 2020 Initiative, 42
Healthy work environments, 14, 41, 73. *See also* Environmental health
High-level wellness, 7
Hispanic theory of disease, 24
HMA, 23, 24
Holistic care
defined, 88
Holistic care, 7
Home health nursing, 34–36
Houses for strangers, 5

I

Illness
defined, 88
Implementation
competencies for, 52, 54–57, 61, 77
coordination of care and, 57
defined, 88
evaluation and, 61
planning and, 52
quality of practice and, 77
standard of practice, 54–56
(2012), 137–138

Infection Control and Emergency
Preparedness Toolkit, 35
Informal learning, 30
Information
defined, 88
on behavior patterns, 19
Intentional care, 1, 3, 4, 10
Intentional care of spirit
defined, 88
Interdisciplinary health care, 29, 36
International Parish Nurse Resource
Center (IPNRC), 4, 7
Internet survey, 42
Interoperability of health information
technology, 39
Interprofessional
defined, 88
Interprofessional collaboration and
teams, 2, 29
competencies for, 46, 50, 54, 55, 57,
64, 66, 67, 70, 72, 76, 80
defined, 88
Interprofessional knowledge and faith
community nursing, 73, 77
Interventions, 3, 12, 21, 27, 32, 34, 36,
37, 43
competencies for, 51–53, 66,
75–76
culturally congruent practice and,
66
evidence-based practice and research
and, 75
outcomes identification and, 51
planning and, 52, 53
quality of practice and, 76
Intervention Scheme (care plans and
services), 11

J

Jameton, Andrew, 14

K

Knowledge, 31
Knowledge, skills, abilities, and judgment
in FCN practice, 25, 26, 29, 31,
47, 72, 74

L

Laws, statutes, and regulations
competencies for, 46, 53, 55, 58, 61,
64, 78, 79
coordination of care and, 58
evidence-based practice and research
and, 78
implementation and, 55
planning and, 53
Leadership, 26, 38. *See also* Spiritual
leader.
collaboration and, 70
communication and, 68
competencies for, 55, 57, 58, 68,
71–72, 77, 80
coordination of care and, 57, 58
implementation and, 55
quality of practice and, 77
resource utilization and, 80
standard of professional performance,
71–72
(2012), 154–155
Learning styles, 42
Legal issues. *See* Laws, statutes, and
regulations
Life transitions, 36–38
Listening, compassionate, 3
Lutheran General Health System, 7

M

Matheus, Rosemarie, 8
Medical appointments, recording of, 22
MEDLINE, 21
Mental health
care, 38
defined, 88–89
Mental illness, 38
Mentoring, 29
Mind–body–spirit components, 3
Minister of health, 27–28
Moral agent
defined, 89
Moral conflicts, 15
Moral distress
defined, 14
Moral resilience
defined, 15

N

National Alliance on Mental Illness (NAMI), 38
National Institutes of Health, 32–33
National Preventive Strategy, 42
New Diagnosis Toolkit, 21
Nightingale, Florence, 6–7
Nontraditional settings, 5
North American Nursing Diagnosis Association (NANDA), 10
Northwest Aging Association, 8
Nurse practitioner, 26, 27
Nurse-led programs, 9
Nurse-to-patient relationship, 13
Nurse-to-profession relationship, 13
Nurse-to-society relationship, 13
Nursing
 defined, 89
Nursing activities. *See* Activities in faith community nursing
Nursing care, 4–5, 7, 10, 12, 27, 31, 39, 55, 71, 75, 76. *See also* Care
Nursing Interventions Classifications and Nursing Outcomes Classifications, 10
Nursing practice
 defined, 89
Nursing process, 15. *See also specific standards*
 defined, 89
 implementation and, 54

O

Omaha System, 10
Organizational policies and procedures, 78
Outcomes, 2, 4, 8, 9, 10, 11, 16, 23, 25, 27, 32, 33, 37, 39. *See also* Evaluation; Outcomes identification; Planning
 collaboration and, 69, 70
 coordination of care and, 57
 culturally congruent practice and, 66
 diagnosis and, 48
 ethics and, 64
 evaluation and, 61

evidence-based practice and research and, 75
 health teaching and health promotion and, 59
 implementation and, 54, 55, 56
 leadership and, 71, 72
 quality of practice and, 76, 77
 resource utilization and, 79
Outcomes identification. *See also* Planning
 competencies for, 50–51
 standard of practice, 50–51
 (2012), 133–134

P

Parish Nurse Resource Center (IPNRC), 7, 8, 28
Parish nurses, 7
Parish nursing, 33
Partnerships, 39, 51, 61, 66, 82
Pastoral associate, 27–28
Patients, 13, 14, 16, 17, 18, 20, 22, 26, 27, 29, 34, 35. *See also* Healthcare consumers
 data, 39
 defined, 89
 education, 37
 evaluation and, 61
 implementation and, 54
 quality of practice and, 76
 spiritual care to, 38
 telehealth use and, 40
Peer review. *See also* Collaboration; Communication
 defined, 89
Plan
 defined, 88
Planning, 10, 24
 competencies for, 52–53, 66
 culturally congruent practice and, 66
 standard of practice, 52–53
 (2012), 135–136
Population
 defined, 89
Population health
 defined, 89
Poverty, 22

T

Technology, 38–40
Telehealth, 79
  forms of, 40
Telemedicine, 40
Theory-driven approaches, 55
Time-limited services, 37
Titling of faith community nurses, 27
Tobacco Free Kids Campaign, 24
Traditional setting, 5
Transitional care
  defined, 91
  models, 37
Trends in faith community nursing,
  33–34, 76

U

Unpaid professional, 40

V

Volunteer, 40
  defined, 91

W

Well-being
  defined, 91
  spiritual, 13, 32, 33

Wellness
  defined, 91
  high-level, 7
    (2012), 118
Wellness diagnoses for health promotion,
  12
Westberg, Granger, 7
Westberg Faith Community Nursing
  Leadership Award, 8
Westberg Institute for Faith Community
  Nursing, 7, 42
Wheat Ridge Foundation, 8
Whole-person care, 1
Whole-person health, 1, 4, 32
  defined, 91
Wholistic
  defined, 91
Wholistic health
  centers, 7
  defined, 7, 91
Wilkerson-Droege Award, 8
Wisconsin model, 8
Work environments, 14, 41, 73. *See also*
  Practice environment.
Work setting. *See* Practice environment.
Workplace safety, 41
Worldview
  defined, 91